Clinical Decision Making and Treatment Planning in Osseointegration

Clinical Decision Making and Treatment Planning in Osseointegration

Michael J. Engelman, DDS

Clinical Associate Professor of Advanced Prosthodontics
Northwestern University Dental School
Chicago, Illinois

Private Practice
Wilmette, Illinois

Quintessence Publishing Co, Inc
Chicago, Berlin, London, Tokyo, São Paulo,
Moscow, Prague, and Warsaw

Dedicated to my wife, Julie

Library of Congress Cataloging-in-Publication Data

Engelman, Michael J.
    Clinical decision making and treatment planning in osseointegration/Michael J. Engelman.
        p.   cm.
    Includes bibliographical references.
    ISBN 0-86715-318-0
    1. Osseointegrated dental implants—Decision making. I. Title.
    [DNLM: 1. Prosthodontics—methods—outlines. 2. Dental Prosthesis—methods—outlines. 3. Dental
Implantation—methods—outlines. 4. Osseointegration—outlines. WU 18.2 E57c 1996]
    RK667.I45E54
    617.6'9—dc20
    DNLM/DLC
    for Library of Congress   96-24841
                                  CIP

 ©1996 by Quintessence Publishing Co, Inc.

Quintessence Publishing Co, Inc
551 N. Kimberly Drive
Carol Stream, IL 60188-1881

Editor: Lane Evensen
Production/Design: Jennifer Sabella
Printing and Binding: Inland Press, WI

Contents

Preface

The purpose of this text is to aid thinking, decision making, and treatment planning in osseointegration. It is intended to be used by the restorative dentist, prosthodontist, and oral surgeon. The clinician may choose to read the book from beginning to end, or may refer to only those sections that apply to the specific patient treated.

The guidelines provided are meant to aid, not restrict. In many instances, the outline can be used as a starting point for discussion, thought, and further research of the literature. The clinician should always remember to treat the entire patient. The bone quality, bone quantity, parafunctional habits, opposing occlusion, maxillomandibular relations, and many other factors all must be included in the decision-making process.

Much of the information has been included here because clinicians in courses have asked questions concerning those topics. An attempt has been made to answer those questions and clarify confusing concepts. Forms have been included to make the thought process and decision making easier for the clinician.

I would like to thank the following individuals for their excellent instruction and guidance during my prosthodontic training: Dr Dennis Barnes, Dr Theodore Berg, Dr John Beumer, Dr Madeline Kurrasch, Dr Steven Lewis, Dr Peter Moy, Dr Arun Sharma, and Dr John Sorensen.

The following individuals have contributed technical instruction and shared invaluable experience that has been included in this manual: Sean Avera, Wayne Mito, Gary Nunakawa, Steve Stevens, and Toshihiro Takasaki.

The lectures and writings of the following individuals have helped with the concepts and ideas presented in this manual: Dr P.-I. Brånemark, Dr Patrick Henry, Dr Torsten Jemt, Dr Steven Lewis, Dr Steve Parel, and Dr Bo Rangert.

The many undergraduate and postgraduate students at UCLA Dental School and Northwestern University School of Dentistry have been a continual stimulus and inspiration to my own dental education. A special thanks to Dr F. J. Kratochvil for introducing me to prosthodontics and allowing me to begin my prosthodontic education. And to Dr John Chai and Dr Richard Sullivan for their assistance in reviewing the text.

Finally, thank you to my father, Dr Joseph Engelman, for his constant optimism and encouragement.

Patient Identification

The patients of a restorative dental practice have been divided into seven categories for convenience. These groups will be used to discuss each situation, the patient's chief complaint and the restorative dental treatment options. The advantages, disadvantages and contraindications of each treatment option will be discussed in this section. There is some repetition between sections. This is intended so that each section may be referred to separately. These same categories are used later in the text to discuss aspects specific to implant restorative dentistry. The categories include:

1. Single Missing Tooth
2. Maxillary Anterior Partially Edentulous
3. Maxillary Posterior Partially Edentulous
4. Mandibular Anterior Partially Edentulous
5. Mandibular Posterior Partially Edentulous
6. Maxillary Completely Edentulous
7. Mandiblular Completely Edentulous

Single Missing Tooth

▼ Situation (Fig 1–1)

1. Esthetic problem due to missing tooth
2. Functional reduction due to missing tooth
3. Risk of eruption of opposing dentition
4. Risk of drift of neighboring teeth
5. Potential for increased risk of caries and periodontal deterioration

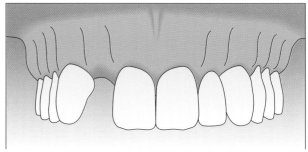

Fig 1-1

▼ Chief Complaint

1. Esthetic problem
2. Functional problem

▼ Treatment Options

1. **Resin-retained fixed partial denture** (Fig 1–2)

   a. Advantages
   1. Less tooth preparation
   2. Fixed prosthesis
   3. Short treatment time
   4. Low patient cost

   b. Disadvantages
   1. Risk of debonding
   2. Risk of sensitivity
   3. Risk of fracture to restoration
   4. Technique sensitivity
   5. Longevity
   6. Esthetics (metal shows through)
   7. Soft-tissue problems under pontic
   8. Compromise of daily maintenance

   c. Contraindications
   1. Significant vertical overlap
   2. High occlusal demands

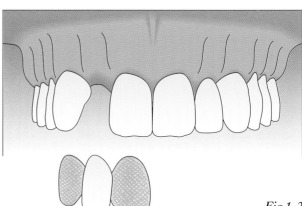

Fig 1-2

2. Fixed partial denture (Fig 1–3)

a. Advantages
1. Predictability
2. Familiarity
3. Fixedness

b. Disadvantages
1. Caries risk
2. Periodontal risk
3. Endodontic risk
4. Risk of cement dissolution
5. Risk of fractured restoration
6. Compromise to daily maintenance
7. Esthetic risk

c. Contraindications
1. Poor abutments
2. Long span
3. Poor abutment placement

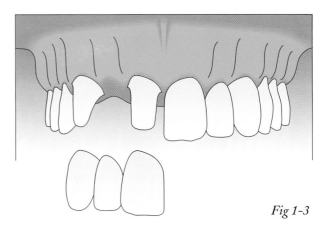

Fig 1-3

3. Removable partial denture (Fig 1–4)

a. Advantages
1. Cost
2. Familiarity

b. Disadvantages
1. Removability
2. Caries risk
3. Periodontal risk
4. Difficulty of adjustment for some patients
5. Need to crown abutments
6. Bulk
7. Speech difficulty
8. Chewing difficulty

c. Contraindication
1. Patient intolerance

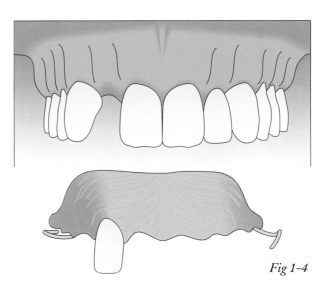

Fig 1-4

4. Implant-supported single crown[1-5]
(Fig 1–5)

a. Advantages
1. No adjacent tooth preparation
2. Accessibility of proximal contacts
3. Absence of caries
4. Bone stabilization
5. Retrievability

b. Disadvantages
1. Limited clinical results
2. Risk of screw loosening
3. Risk of restoration fracture
4. Risk of fixture failure
5. Inability to replace missing interdental papilla
6. Visibility of metal through tissue
7. Length of treatment time
8. Risk of cement dissolution
9. Need for surgery

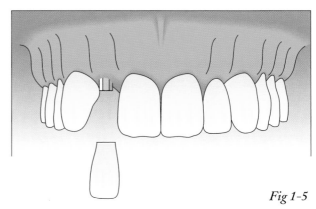

Fig 1-5

c. Contraindications
1. Avoided by some clinicians for:
   a. Canine
   b. Deep vertical overlap
   c. First molar
   d. Mandibular incisors limited mesiodistal (dimensions)
2. Medical contraindications
   a. Pregnancy
   b. Inability of patient to have elective surgery
   c. Other conditions

5. Other solutions

a. Orthodontics

Maxillary Anterior— Partially Edentulous

▼ Situation (Fig 1–6)

1. Esthetic problem due to missing teeth
2. Functional problem due to missing teeth
3. Risk of eruption of opposing dentition
4. Risk of drifting of neighboring teeth
5. Future potential increased risk of caries and periodontal breakdown

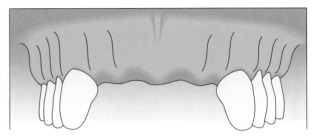

Fig 1-6

▼ Chief Complaint

1. Esthetic problem
2. Functional problem

▼ Treatment Options

1. Fixed partial denture (Fig 1–7)

a. Advantages
1. Fixedness
2. Predictability
3. Familiarity
4. Longevity

b. Disadvantages
1. Caries risk
2. Endodontic risk
3. Periodontal risk
4. Risk of restoration fracture
5. Risks associated with longevity
6. Risk of cement dissolution

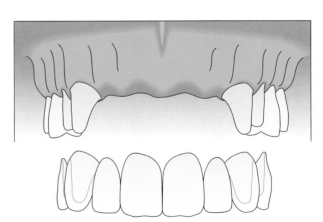

Fig 1-7

c. Contraindications
1. Inadequate abutments
2. Excessive anterior-posterior span of fixed partial denture from abutment to labial surface
3. Inadequate abutment placement

2. Removable partial denture (Fig 1–8)

a. Advantages
1. Cost to patient
2. Familiarity
3. Ability to replace lost teeth and ridge

b. Disadvantages
1. Bulk
2. Removability
3. Caries risk
4. Periodontal risk
5. Need for crowns on abutments (for denture insertion and removal)
6. Speech difficulty
7. Taste alteration
8. Palatal coverage discomfort for some patients
9. Difficulty of achieving esthetic needs for some patients

c. Contraindication
1. Patient intolerance

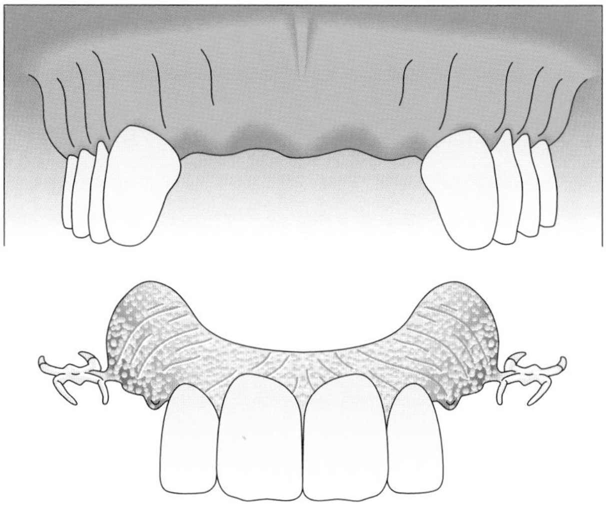

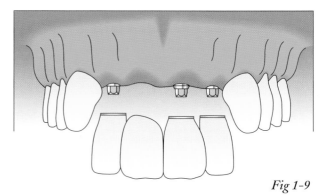

Fig 1-8

3. Implant-supported fixed partial denture (Fig 1–9)

a. Advantages
1. Improvement of function
2. Fixedness
3. Retrievability
4. Bone stability
5. No need for tooth preparation

Fig 1-9

b. Disadvantages
1. Risk of restoration fracture
2. Risk of screw fracture
3. Risk of screw loosening
4. Need for two surgeries
5. Length of treatment time
6. Possibility of implant fracture or failure
7. Challenging esthetics

c. Contraindications
1. Inadequate bone at anticipated implant site
   a. Inadequate vertical bone height
   b. Inadequate bone width
   c. Excessive bony concavities
   d. These are all relative contraindications as surgical procedures can often be performed to solve them
2. Inadequate vertical space for prosthesis
3. Medical contraindications
   a. Pregnancy
   b. Inability to have elective surgery
   c. Other conditions

Maxillary Posterior— Partially Edentulous

▼ Situation (Fig 1–10)

1. Functional problem due to missing teeth
2. Esthetic problem due to missing teeth for some patients
3. Risk of eruption of opposing dentition
4. Risk of drift of neighboring teeth
5. Possible increased caries and periodontal breakdown
6. Lack of posterior support, which may jeopardize muscular and temporo-mandibular joint comfort

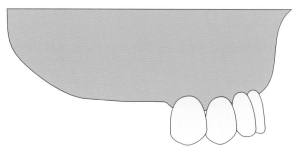

Fig 1-10

▼ Chief Complaint

1. Functional problem
2. Esthetic problem

▼ Treatment Options

1. Removable partial denture (Fig 1–11)

   a. Advantages
   1. Cost
   2. Familiarity
   3. Replaces missing posterior support
   4. Prevents supereruption of opposing teeth
   5. Ease of daily maintenance
   6. Restores missing hard and soft tissues

   b. Disadvantages
   1. Difficulty with speech
   2. Removability
   3. Bone resorption under tissue-borne extension
   4. Jeopardy to remaining tooth

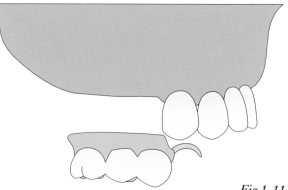

Fig 1-11

8
▼

5. Caries risk
6. Periodontal risk
7. Needed for abutment preparation
8. Difficulty of adapting for some patients
9. Prosthesis wear and risk of fracture
10. Adjustment period
11. Soft-tissue irritation
12. Must crown some teeth to make placement possible

c. Contraindication
1. Patient intolerance

2. **Fixed partial denture with cantilevered pontic (no posterior abutment)** (Fig 1–12)
   a. Advantages
   1. Fixedness
   2. Familiarity

   b. Disadvantages
   1. Risk of cement dissolution
   2. Caries risk
   3. Endodontic risk
   4. Periodontal risk
   5. Risk of fracture restoration
   6. Longevity

   c. Contraindication
   1. Inadequate abutments

3. **Fixed partial denture (with posterior abutment)** (Fig 1–13)
   a. Advantages
   1. Fixedness
   2. Familiarity

   b. Disadvantages
   1. Caries risk
   2. Risk of cement dissolution
   3. Periodontal risk

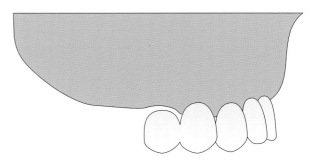

Fig 1-12

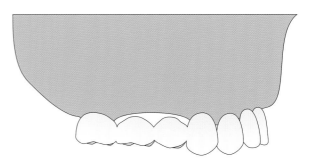

Fig 1-13

Fixed partial denture (with posterior abutment)/Disadvantages (continued)

4. Endodontic risk
5. Risk of fractured restoration
6. Longevity
7. Esthetic risk

c. Contraindications
1. Inadequate abutments
2. Excessive span

4. Implant-supported fixed partial denture[6-20] (Fig 1–14)

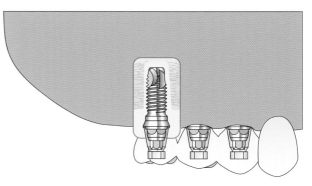

Fig 1-14

a. Advantages
1. Fixedness
2. Retrievability
3. Independence from natural teeth
4. Bone stability

b. Disadvantages
1. Risk of screw loosening
2. Risk of screw fracture
3. Possibility of implant fracture or failure
4. Need for two surgeries
5. Length of treatment time
6. Risk of restoration fracture

c. Contraindications
1. Inadequate bone at anticipated implant site
   (Note: This is a relative contra-indication and can often be overcome by surgical procedures.)
   a. Inadequate vertical height of bone inferior to the maxillary sinus
   b. Poor quality of bone at site
2. Medical contraindications
   a. Pregnancy
   b. Inability to have elective surgery
   c. Other conditions

Mandibular Anterior— Partially Edentulous

▼ Situation (Fig 1–15)

1. Esthetic problem due to missing teeth
2. Functional problem due to missing teeth
3. Risk of eruption of opposing dentition
4. Risk of drift of neighboring teeth
5. Future increased caries and periodontal risks

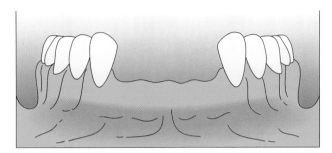

Fig 1-15

▼ Chief Complaint

1. Poor esthetics
2. Poor function

▼ Treatment Options (Fig 1–16)

1. Fixed partial denture

a. Advantages
1. Familiarity
2. Fixedness

b. Disadvantages
1. Need for tooth preparation
2. Caries risk
3. Endodontic risk
4. Periodontal risk
5. Risk of restoration fracture
6. Risk of cement dissolution

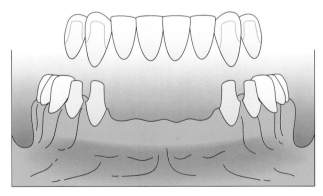

Fig 1-16

c. Contraindications
1. Inadequate abutments
2. Excessive span

2. Removable partial denture (Fig 1–17)

a. Advantage
1. Cost to patient
2. Familiarity
3. Ability to replace lost ridge and teeth

b. Disadvantages
1. Bulk
2. Removability
3. Speech difficulty
4. Necessary to extend posteriorly
5. Caries risk
6. Periodontal risk
7. Necessary to crown abutment teeth

c. Contraindication
1. Patient intolerance

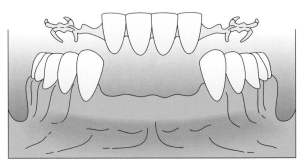

Fig 1-17

3. Implant-supported fixed partial denture[6-20] (Fig 1–18)

a. Advantages
1. Fixedness
2. Retrievability
3. Improved function
4. No tooth preparation
5. No caries risk
6. Predictable success in mandibular anterior region
7. Bone stabilization

b. Disadvantages
1. Risk of screw loosening
2. Risk of screw fracture
3. Possibility of implant loss
4. Need for two surgeries
5. Length of treatment time
6. Risk of restoration fracture

c. Contraindication
1. Medical contraindications
   a. Pregnancy
   b. Inability to have elective surgery
   c. Other medical conditions

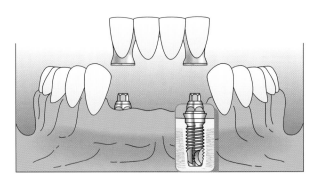

Fig 1-18

Mandibular Posterior— Partially Edentulous

▼ Situation (Fig 1–19)

1. Functional problem due to missing teeth
2. Risk of eruption of opposing dentition
3. Lack of posterior support, which may jeopardize muscular and temporomandibular joint comfort
4. Future increased caries and periodontal risks

▼ Chief Complaint

1. Functional problem due to missing teeth
2. Patient unable to function with existing removable prosthesis

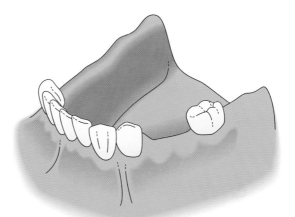

Fig 1-19

▼ Treatment Options

1. Removable partial denture (Fig 1–20)

a. Advantages
   1. Familiarity
   2. Low cost to the patient

b. Disadvantages
   1. Removability
   2. Bulk
   3. Speech difficulty
   4. Function loss
   5. Difficulty chewing
   6. Continued bone resorption under prosthesis
   7. Need to crown abutments

c. Contraindication
   1. Not acceptable to patient
   2. Length of treatment time
   3. Need for two surgeries

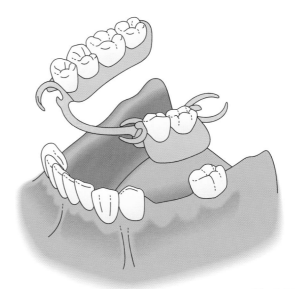

Fig 1-20

2. Fixed partial denture with cantilevered pontic (no posterior abutment)
(Fig 1–21)

a. Advantage
1. Fixed prosthesis

b. Disadvantages
1. Risk of dissolution of cement
2. Risk of partial denture fracture
3. Possibility of periodontal loss due to excessive load on tooth
4. Caries risk
5. Endodontic risk
6. Periodontal risk

c. Contraindication
1. Abutments inadequate to fabricate restoration

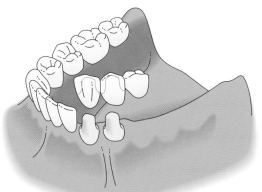

Fig 1-21

3. Fixed partial denture (with posterior abutment) (Fig 1–22)

a. Advantages
1. Familiarity
2. Predictability

b. Disadvantages
1. Caries risk
2. Periodontal risk
3. Endodontic risk
4. Risk of restoration fracture
5. Risk of cement dissolution

c. Contraindications
1. Excessive span
2. Inadequate abutments

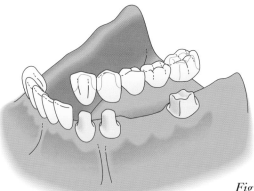

Fig 1-22

4. Implant-supported fixed partial denture[6-20] (Fig 1–23)

a. Advantages

1. Fixedness
2. Retrievability
3. Bone stabilization
4. No tooth preparation of adjacent teeth
5. No caries risk
6. Improved function

b. Disadvantages

1. Risk of screw loosening
2. Risk of screw fracture
3. Possibility of implant loss
4. Need for two surgeries
5. Length of treatment time
6. Risk of restoration fracture

c. Contraindication

1. Inadequate bone above the inferior alveolar nerve canal

   (Note: This is a relative contraindication as surgical procedures can solve problem.)
2. Medical contraindications
   a. Pregnancy
   b. Inability to have elective surgery
   c. Other conditions

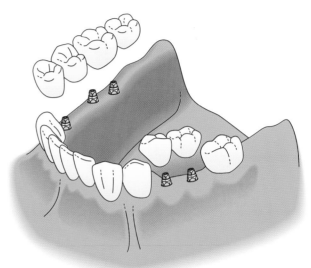

Fig 1-23

Maxilla—Completely Edentulous

▼ Situation
1. Completely edentulous arch (Fig 1–24)
2. Continued resorption of maxilla beneath complete denture prosthesis
3. Combination syndrome

   There is often severe resorption of the anterior maxilla for patients with retained mandibular anterior teeth. This reduces the chance of success with a conventional prosthesis.

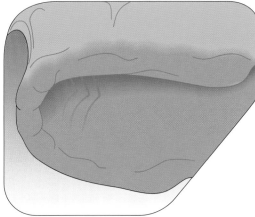

Fig 1-24

▼ Chief Complaint
1. Patient unable to tolerate existing prosthesis
   a. Palatal coverage is a problem
   b. Altered taste sensations
   c. Loose maxillary complete denture
   d. Psychological inability to wear
   e. Patient dislikes removable aspect of prosthesis

▼ Treatment Options

1. Complete denture (Fig 1–25)

a. Advantages
1. Familiarity
2. Cost
3. Predictability
4. Tolerated well by most patients
5. Restores missing teeth

b. Disadvantages
1. Bone resorption
2. Removability
3. Low occlusal bite force
4. Speech problems
5. Taste problems
6. Longevity
7. Palatal coverage
8. Gag problems
9. Multiple adjustments
10. Soft-tissue conditioners necessary
11. Risk of denture fracture
12. Instability
13. Non-retentiveness

c. Contraindication
1. Patient inability to wear prosthesis

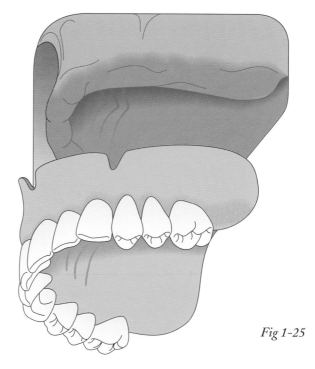

Fig 1-25

2. Subperiosteal implant

a. Advantage
1. Increased stability of prosthesis

b. Disadvantages
1. Bone resorption under implant
2. Lack of predictable long-term success

c. Contraindication
1. This treatment option should be avoided in the maxilla due to its poor bone quality. Some patients have significant resorption under the sub-periosteal implant in the maxilla.

3. Implant-supported overdenture[21,22,24,26,28]
(Fig 1–26)

a. Advantages
1. Removability
2. Access for maintenance
3. Control of profile and facial contours
4. Increased stability
5. Increased retention
6. Increased bite force
7. Improved proprioception
8. Psychological improvement
9. Retrievability
10. Speech similar to what can be accomplished with a maxillary complete denture

b. Disadvantages
1. Risk of screw fracture
2. Risk of screw loosening
3. Possibility of implant failure
4. Risk of denture fracture
5. Risk of denture tooth fracture
6. Length of treatment time
7. Need for two surgeries
8. Need for maintenance (of retentive components and denture)
9. Need for adjustment

c. Contraindications
1. Inadequate bone to place adequate number of implants
2. Medical contraindications
   a. Pregnancy
   b. Patient inability to undergo elective surgery
   c. Other medical conditions

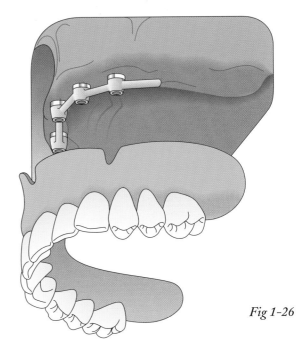

Fig 1-26

4. Implant-supported fixed partial denture[26-30] (Fig 1–27)

a. Advantages
1. Fixedness
2. Retrievability
3. Longevity
4. Predictability
5. Increased stability
6. Increased retention
7. Bone stabilization

b. Disadvantages
1. Speech problems (air escape)
2. Hygiene maintenance problems
3. Esthetic problem with short lip and high smile
4. Possibility of implant failure
5. Risk of screw fracture
6. Risk of screw loosening
7. Risk of prosthesis fracture
8. Length of treatment time
9. Need for two surgeries
10. Risk of prosthetic tooth fracture

c. Contraindications
1. Too little bone to place adequate number of implants
2. Medical contraindications
   a. Pregnancy
   b. Inability to tolerate elective surgery
   c. Other medical conditions

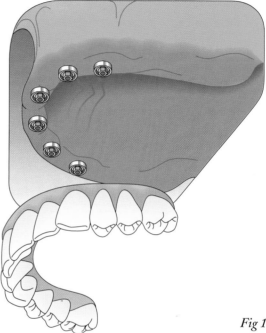

Fig 1-27

Mandible—Completely Edentulous

▼ Situation

1. Arch is completely edentulous (Fig 1–28)
2. Mucosa is often thin and non-keratinized
3. Resorption of mandible continues under existing complete denture
4. Floor of the mouth is often higher than residual ridge
5. Mental nerve and inferior alveolar bone superior to the nerve

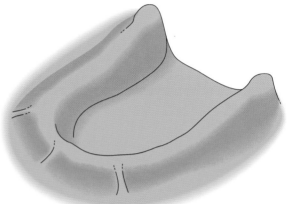

Fig 1-28

▼ Chief Complaint

1. Inability to chew
2. Painful chewing
3. Loose existing complete denture
4. Need to remove prosthesis
5. Psychological inability to tolerate existing prosthesis

▼ Treatment Options

1. Complete denture (Fig 1–29)

   a. Advantages
   1. Familiarity
   2. Cost

   b. Disadvantages
   1. Removability
   2. Possible tissue soreness
   3. Poor function
   4. Poor speech
   5. Poor chewing
   6. Longevity
   7. Continued bone resorption

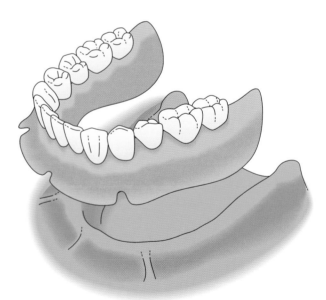

Fig 1-29

8. Financial loss leader for many dentists
9. Loss of interarch distance
10. High maintenance due to multiple adjustments
11. Soft-tissue conditioners necessary

2. Vestibuloplasty and skin graft

a. Advantages
1. Increased bearing surface
2. Increased keratinized surface
3. Patient acceptance

b. Disadvantages
1. Need for surgery
2. Hair growth of graft
3. Sebaceous gland activity of graft
4. Altered taste sensations
5. Still removable prosthesis
6. Two surgical sites

c. Contraindication
1. Patient intolerance

3. Augmentation of mandible

a. Advantages
1. Increased vertical height of residual ridge
2. Increased bearing surface

b. Disadvantages
1. Limited longevity
2. Resorption of graft
3. High-maintenance prosthesis
4. Constant need for soft-tissue conditioners and adjustments
5. Two surgical sites

4. Hydroxylapatite augmentation

a. Advantages
1. One surgical site
2. Increased bearing surface
3. Increased vertical height of ridge

b. Disadvantages
1. Lack of long-term clinical studies
2. Changing bearing surface
3. Movement of material
4. Risk of losing material through tissue perforation
5. Risk of material moving into mental-nerve region (causing parasthesia, anesthesia or altered sensation)
6. Pain

5. Subperiosteal implant-supported denture

a. Advantages
1. Stable prosthesis
2. Increased occlusal bite force

b. Disadvantages
1. Lack of long-term predictable results
2. Risk of implant fracture
3. Risk of bone loss around implant
4. Possibility of soft-tissue problems around post
5. Limited longevity
6. Need for two surgical procedures with techniques

6. Ramus frame implant

a. Advantage
1. Increased stability and retention of prosthesis

b. Disadvantages
1. Unpredictability
2. Lack of vertical space for prosthesis above ramus frame
3. Risk of bone loss around implant
4. Need for surgical placement

7. Implant-supported overdenture[21-24,31-33]

(Fig 1–30)

a. Advantages

1. Removability
2. Hygiene access
3. Similarity to patient's complete denture
4. Cost
5. Retrievability
6. Profile and external contour control
7. Increased occlusal bite force
8. Improved patient confidence and psychological aspects
9. Ease of fabrication for patient with difficult maxillo-mandibular relations
10. Increased retention of prosthesis
11. Increased stability of prosthesis
12. Implants placed in a predictable region (the anterior mandible)
13. Improved proprioception
14. Anterior bone stabilization

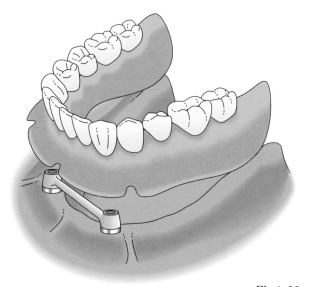

Fig 1-30

b. Disadvantages

1. Need for adjustments
2. Continued bone resorption in posterior region
3. Need for maintenance of prosthesis
   a. Soft-tissue conditioners
   b. Adjustments
   c. Denture repairs
   d. Replacement or repair of retentive component
4. Length of treatment time
5. Need for two surgeries
6. Potential bone resorption of the opposing (anterior) completely edentulous maxilla

c. Contraindications

1. Inadequate bone for implant placement (rare)
2. Medical contraindications
   a. Pregnancy
   b. Inability to undergo elective surgery
   c. Other medical conditions

8. Implant-supported fixed prosthesis[26-30]
(Fig 1–31)

a. Advantages
1. Predictability
2. Fixedness
3. Retrievability
4. No compressive force on mandible
5. Improved function
6. Increased bite force
7. Increased proprioception
8. Reduced resorption of the mandible
9. Lower maintenance of prosthesis
10. Increased stability of prosthesis
11. Increased retention of prosthesis
12. Long-term published clinical success
13. Bone stabilization

b. Disadvantages
1. Need for two surgeries
2. Risk of screw loosening
3. Risk of screw fracture
4. Risk of restoration fracture
5. Possibility of implant failure
6. Length of treatment time
7. Maintenance and recall commitment
8. Inability of some patients to perform daily oral hygiene procedures around prosthesis and components
9. Potential bone resorption of the opposing edentulous maxilla

c. Contraindications
1. Too little bone for adequate number of implants
2. Medical contraindications
   a. Pregnancy
   b. Inability to undergo elective surgery
   c. Other medical conditions

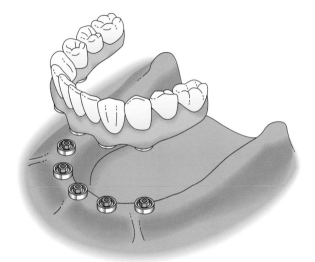

Fig 1-31

References

▼ Single Missing Tooth

1. Schmitt A, Zarb G. The longitudinal and clinical effectiveness of osseointegrated dental implants for single tooth replacement. Int J Prosthodont 1993;6:197–202.

2. Laney W, Jemt T, Harris D, et al. Osseointegrated implants for single tooth replacement: Progress report from a multicenter prospective study after 3 years. Int J Oral Maxillofac Implants 1994;9:49–54.

3. Ekfeldt A, Carlsson G, Borjesson G. Clinical evaluation of single tooth restorations supported by osseointegrated implants: A retrospective study. Int J Oral Maxillofac Implants 1994;9:179–183.

4. Jemt T, Lekholm U, Grondahl. A 3-year follow-up study of early single implant restorations add modum Brånemark. Int J Periodont Rest Dent 1990;10:341–349.

5. Andersson B, Ödman P, Carlsson L, et al. A new Brånemark single tooth abutment: handling and early clinical experiences. Int J Oral Maxillofac Implants 1992;7:105–111.

▼ Partially Edentulous

6. Henry P, Tolman D, Bolender C. The applicability of osseointegrated implants in the treatment of partially edentulous patients: Three-year results of a prospective multicenter study. Quintessence Int 1993;24:123–129.

7. Naert I, Quirynen M, Van Steenberghe D, Darius P. A six-year prosthodontic study of 509 consecutively inserted implants for the treatment of partial edentulism. J Prosthet Dent 1992;67:236–245.

8. Nevins M, Langer B. The successful application of osseointegrated implants to the posterior jaw: A long-term retrospective study. Int J Oral Maxillofac Implants 1993;8:428–432.

9. Bahat O. Treatment planning and placement of implants in the posterior maxillae: Report of 732 consecutive Nobelpharma implants. Int J Oral Maxillofac Implants 1993;8:151–161.

10. Drago C. Rates of osseointegration of dental implants with regard to anatomical location. J Prosthod 1992;1:29–31.

11. Ericsson I, Brånemark PI, Glantz DO. Partial edentulism. In: Worthington P, Brånemark PI, eds. Advanced Osseointegration Surgery: Applications in the Maxillofacial Region. Chicago: Quintessence; 1992:194–209.

12. Van Steenburghe D, Lekholm U, Bolender C, et al. The applicability of osseointegrated oral implants in the rehabilitation of partial edentulism: A prospective multicenter study on 558 fixtures. Int J Oral Maxillofac Implants 1990;5:272–281.

13. Van Steenburghe D. A retrospective multicenter evaluation of the survival rate of osseointegrated fixtures supporting fixed partial prostheses in the treatment of partial edentulism. J Prosthet Dent 1989;61:217–223.

14. Pylant T, Triplett G, Key M, Brunsvold M. A retrospective evaluation of endosseous titanium implants in the partially edentulous patient. Int J Oral Maxillofac Implants 1992;7:195–202.

15. Bahat O. Osseointegrated implants in the maxillary tuberosity: report on 45 consecutive patients. Int J Oral Maxillofac Implants 1992;7:459–467.

16. Zarb G, Schmitt A. The longitudinal clinical effectiveness of osseointegrated dental implants in anterior partially edentulous patients. Int J Prosthodont 1993;6:180–188.

17. Zarb G, Schmitt A. The longitudinal clinical effectiveness of osseointegrated dental implants in posterior partially edentulous patients. Int J Prosthodont 1993;6:189–196.

18. Jemt T, Lekholm U, Adell R. Osseointegrated implants in the treatment of partially edentulous patients: A preliminary study on 876 consecutively placed fixtures. Int J Oral Maxillofac Implants 1989;4:211–217.

19. Jemt T, Linden B, Lekholm U. Failures and complications in 127 consecutively placed fixed partial prostheses supported by Brånemark implants: From prosthetic treatment to first annual checkup. Int J Oral Maxillofac Implants 1992;7:40–44.

20. Jemt T, Lekholm U. Oral implant treatment in posterior partially edentulous jaws: A 5-year follow-up report. Int J Oral Maxillofac Implants 1993;8:635–640.

▼ Completely Edentulous

21. Johns RB, Jemt T, Heath M, et al. A multicenter study of overdentures supported by Brånemark implants. Int J Oral Maxillofac Implants 1992;7:513–522.

22. Naert I, Quirynen M, Theuniers G, et al. Prosthetic aspects of osseointegrated fixtures supporting overdentures. A 4-year report. J Prosthet Dent 1991;65:671–680.

23. Tolman D, Laney W. Tissue integrated prosthesis complications. Int J Oral Maxillofac Implants 1992;7:477–484.

24. Engquist B, Bergendal T, Kallus T, Linden V. A retrospective multicenter evaluation of osseointegrated implants supporting overdentures. Int J Oral Maxillofac Implants 1988;3:129–134.

25. Jemt T, Book K, Linden B, Urde G. Failures and complications in 92 consecutively inserted overdentures supported by Brånemark implants in severely resorbed edentulous maxilla: A study from prosthetic treatment to first annual checkup. Int J Oral Maxillofac Implants 1992;7:162–167.

26. Adell R, Eriksson B, Lekholm U, et al. A long-term follow-up study of osseointegrated implants in the treatment of totally edentulous jaws. Int J Oral Maxillofac Implants 1990;5:347–359.

27. Zarb G, Schmitt A. The longitudinal clinical effectiveness of osseointegrated dental implants: The Toronto study. Part III: Problems and complications encountered. J Prosthet Dent 1990;64:185–194.

28. Friberg B, Jemt T, Lekholm U. Early failures in 4,641 consecutively placed Brånemark dental implants: A study from stage I surgery to the connection of completed prostheses. Int J Oral Maxillofac Implants 1991;6:142–146.

29. Jemt T. Failures and complications in 391 consecutively inserted fixed prostheses supported by Brånemark implants in edentulous jaws: A study of treatment from the time of prosthetic placement to the first annual checkup. Int J Oral Maxillofac Implants 1991;6:270–276.

30. Adell R, Lekholm U, Rockler B, et al. A 15-year study of osseointegrated implants in the treatment of the edentulous jaw. Int J Oral Surg 1981;10:387–416.

31. Triplett G, Mason M, Alfonso W, et al. Endosseous cylinder implants in severely atrophic mandibles. Int J Oral Maxillofac Implants 1991;6:264–269.

32. Hennys K, Schmitt A, Zarb G. Complications and maintenance requirements for fixed prostheses and overdentures in the edentulous mandible: A 5-year report. Int J Oral Maxillofac Implants 1994;9;191–196.

33. Naert I, DeClercq M, Theuniers G, Schepers E. Overdentures supported by osseointegrated fixtures for the edentulous mandible: A 2.5 year report. Int J Oral Maxillofac Implants 1988;3:191–196.

Patient Education

Educating patients regarding implant restorative dentistry is critical. This section lists several of the tools available to the clinician and staff to inform the patient. Each clinician may select those techniques that best assist the patient in understanding the treatment options and how implants can accomplish the established goals.

The dental staff is very useful in assisting the restorative dentist in educating the potential patient about implants. The receptionist, dental assistant, and dental hygienist can often educate the patient about the benefits of implants. The dental auxiliaries should be encouraged to attend continuing education programs concerning dental implants to expand their own knowledge base. The auxiliaries often have innovative suggestions on how to help patients understand concepts.

Casts

1. Several casts are available with removable components intended for patient education.
2. Casts from previous patients are often useful in illustrating a specific clinical situation.

Video

1. Show to patient in office.
2. Loan to patient.

Photographic Documentation of Own Patients

1. Assemble book of treated-patient photos.
2. Slides of patient examples can be arranged in a slide carousel and patients can view these in the clinician's office.

Completed Patients

1. Previously treated patients can be contacted to talk with potential implant patients concerning their implant experience.
2. Some offices contact the completed patient to confirm availability to talk with a potential implant patient. These offices will give the completed patient the phone number of the potential patient. The completed patient will then contact the new patient.

What Patients Should Know at Consultation Appointment

Some clinicians keep this discussion short and concise. Other clinicians delegate this responsibility to an auxiliary or implant coordinator.

1. Treatment planning phase
   a. Surgical consultation
   b. Restorative-surgical planning
   c. Use of surgical guide
   d. Radiographs
   e. Short discussion
2. Time explanation: two-stage surgery with long-term commitment
   a. Implants placed at first surgery
   b. Period of healing-osseointegration
      1. mandible: 4 months (minimum)
      2. maxilla: 6 months (minimum)
   c. Implants uncovered at second surgery
   d. Soft-tissue healing: 2–8 weeks
   e. Restorative appointments: 1–3 months
3. Maintenance and regular recall
   a. Regular prophylaxis and examination
   b. Daily maintenance commitment
   c. Office repair and replacement policy
4. Fee and payment policy
   a. Total estimated restorative fee should be listed
   b. Office payment policy
      1. Monthly payments
      2. Payments in thirds
         • one-third as treatment begins
         • one-third at final impression appointment
         • final third at delivery appointment
      3. Other options

Tracking Implant Patients

2

1. Implant coordinator
   a. Some offices will appoint an implant coordinator whose responsibilities include:
      1. Follow-up of patients who have had an implant consultation
      2. Tracking patients as they proceed through the series of appointments
      3. Assuring that completed restorative patients are included in a reevaluation, reexamination, and maintenance schedule
2. Implant patient tracking form (see form page 30)
   a. Needed appointments
   b. Patient's standing in sequence of appointments
      1. Treatment planning checklist
      2. Restorative/surgical consultation
      3. First surgery: implant placed
      4. Adjustment of temporary prosthesis
      5. Second surgery: implant uncovered, healing abutment placed
      6. Definitive abutment placed
      7. Restorative procedures list
      8. Insertion of prosthesis
      9. Reevaluation at one week
      10. Maintenance and recall

Implant Patient Tracking Form

Patient	Restorative Consultation	Surgical Consultation	Laboratory Consultation	Joint Consultation	Stent	Preprosthetic Surgery	1st Surgery Implant Placement	Adjust Prosthesis	2nd Surgery Implant Uncovered	Abutment Selection	Definitive Abutment Connection	Provisionals	Prosthetic Procedures	Prosthesis Delivery	1-week Re-evaluation	Recall & Maintenance
1.																
2.																
3.																
4.																
5.																
6.																
7.																
8.																
9.																
10.																
11.																
12.																
13.																
14.																
15.																
16.																
17.																
18.																
19.																
20.																
21.																
22.																
23.																
24.																
25.																

Treatment Planning Letter

This letter (pages 32–33) is prepared for the patient after the treatment plan has been established but prior to implant placement. It informs the patient about his or her existing dental condition and the planned treatment.

1. Problem list (existing conditions detailed in sentence form)
   a. Maxilla
   b. Mandible
   c. Diagnosis
2. Treatment options
   a. Advantages
   b. Disadvantages
   c. Prognosis
3. Financial discussion
   a. Estimated restorative fee
   b. Note does not include surgical fee
   c. Payment policy
   d. Policy if there are changes in treatment plan or fee
   e. Maintenance fee/repair fee/policy
   f. Adjustment policy

Treatment Information Forms

1. Further description of restorative options
   a. For the single missing tooth (pages 34–36)
   b. For multiple missing teeth (pages 37–38)
   c. For the edentulous maxilla (pages 39–41)
   d For the edentulous mandible (pages 42–43)
2. Explanation of available procedures using osseointegrated implants
3. Intended for patient education
   a. To help the patient weigh the options (if given at the initial visit)
   b. To help the patient understand the treatment plan (if given with the treatment planning letter)

2

▼ Treatment Planning Letter

Dear Patient:

At your recent consultation appointment, we discussed those procedures necessary to restore your mouth to optimal dental health. To be sure that you have complete understanding of the procedures to be undertaken, I would like to outline the information that we discussed.

As you know, your upper teeth have been replaced by a complete denture. Your existing complete denture is loose and unstable. Several of the teeth are fractured and stained.

In your lower arch, you have an existing removable partial denture that has fractured and been repaired several times. You also have six remaining teeth: 22 through 27. Teeth 22 and 27 have decay encircling the entire edge of the crown. All six remaining teeth have lost more than one half of the supporting bone surrounding them.

We discussed your options for your upper jaw and you have elected to have a new upper complete denture. Implants and a prosthesis may be placed in your upper jaw at a later date if you desire.

As in any complex restorative treatment plan, you have several options for your lower jaw. One option would be to retain your remaining mandibular anterior teeth; crown all of these teeth and fabricate a new removable partial denture. This is not a recommended option because of the poor prognosis of your teeth.

Your second option would be to fabricate a lower immediate complete denture and remove all of your remaining natural teeth. The disadvantage of the immediate denture is that it would be less stable than your current status.

Your final option is the option that you and I have discussed, and in which you have expressed interest. This would involve removal of all your remaining mandibular teeth, including teeth 22 and 27. On the same day that these are removed by your oral surgeon, our office would deliver to you a mandibular immediate complete denture. This would be adjusted for several months. After healing of the soft tissue and bone has completed, your oral surgeon would place five osseointegrated implants in your lower jaw. This would be followed by a minimum healing period of four months, and then a second surgery would uncover the implants. After a short period of soft-tissue or gum-tissue healing, our office would then fabricate a fixed prosthesis that would be supported by your implants.

2

The advantage of this treatment is that you have an option that has a predictable rate of success. Another advantage of this option is that the prosthesis will be retrievable (removable) if the need arises. It is only removable by a dentist. With this treatment plan we have solved your missing teeth problem; esthetics are controlled and can be adjusted to fulfill your requirements. This is a fixed partial denture that you do not have to remove on a daily basis.

One disadvantage of this option is that the teeth on the biting surface of the prosthesis may occasionally wear out and need replacing (whereas with your removable partial denture occasional reliners were needed). A second disadvantage is that during the healing period you will be wearing a complete denture. Some of our patients find that this is a challenging time during their treatment because they have a denture that is resting entirely on the gum tissue.

The estimated fee for your restorative procedure is $_____. This fee includes a mandibular immediate complete denture, a maxillary complete denture, a mandibular fixed partial denture on implants, and adjusting the prostheses for two months after delivery. If any additional appointments are necessary after this two month adjustment period, there will be an additional fee based on the amount of time and materials required. These are the fees for restorative procedures completed at our office and do not include any surgical fees for procedures completed by your surgeon.

In our office we ask that our patients pay at the time of service, with final payment due upon placement of the final restorations. As you know, in any complex treatment plan, there are occasional changes in the anticipated treatment. If there is a change in plan or fee our office will notify you.

I look forward to working with you and I appreciate you seeking your dental care in our office. If you have any questions please contact me.

Sincerely,

I have read and understand the above information:

Date: _____ Name: _____

Signature: _____

Information Concerning the Single Missing Tooth

People who have lost a single tooth face a special type of problem. Esthetics or appearance usually motivate the individual to replace the tooth, but the continual natural development and movement of the other teeth make replacement especially important. If nothing is done to replace the missing tooth there is a risk of movement of the teeth in the opposite jaw, and also a risk of neighboring teeth drifting into the space. The simple fact that there is one less tooth for the person to chew on reduces chewing ability.

Fortunately, there are several restorative options that a patient may choose to replace a single missing tooth. The restorative options include a resin-retained partial denture, a fixed partial denture, a removable partial denture, or an implant-supported single crown. There are advantages and disadvantages to each of these options.

The nature of these treatments, as well as their advantages and disadvantages, are described below. This information is designed to help you understand the treatment options now available.

Option 1—Fixed Partial Denture

In this procedure the teeth on either side of the space are prepared or shaped. A fixed partial denture of metal or metal and porcelain, which includes the replacement tooth, is then cemented on the neighboring teeth. The disadvantage of this option is that there is a risk of decay on the teeth and possible nerve damage. There is a risk to the gum tissue and the bone surrounding the teeth, which may lead to periodontal problems. Some partial dentures become uncemented and occasionally fracture. Daily cleaning is difficult with some partial dentures. There is also an esthetic risk because the goal of this restoration is to match the remaining teeth, which often proves challenging. A fixed partial denture cannot be used on teeth that do not have enough bone surrounding them or enough tooth structure to hold the length of the partial denture in place.

The advantage to this treatment method is familiarity; both cost and outcome are predictable. A fixed partial denture replaces the missing tooth, stabilizes the bite, and prevents movement of opposing teeth.

2

Option 2—Resin-Retained Partial Denture

A resin-retained partial denture is a metal and porcelain replacement of the missing tooth. The restoration is cemented to the back side of the adjacent teeth. Like a conventional fixed partial denture, a resin-retained partial denture is fixed or non-removable. However, this type of partial denture requires less tooth preparation. It replaces the missing tooth, stabilizes the bite, and prevents movement of opposing teeth. While the treatment time of completion is very short, this option does have several disadvantages. There is a risk of loosening or debonding in many patients. There is also risk of sensitivity of the tooth or fracture of the restoration. The longevity of this restoration is also variable. Occasionally, metal shows through on the adjacent teeth and esthetics are compromised. Sometimes, there is a soft-tissue problem underneath the partial denture when daily cleaning is difficult. This option is often selected for very young patients and some dentists consider it a temporary restoration until they are older. Then one of the other definitive restorations is placed.

Option 3—Removable Partial Denture

This is a removable prosthesis fabricated out of metal, acrylic, and denture teeth for the patient. The disadvantage of this option is that it jeopardizes many of the surrounding teeth, resulting in a risk of decay and gum tissue problems. Some patients have difficulty adjusting to the prosthesis. They find speech and chewing difficult. These patients often find this prosthesis very bulky. For some, it is necessary to crown or contour teeth in order to be able to insert and remove the partial denture. In some situations, there is metal that holds the partial in place, but is visible when the patient smiles. It can, however, be uncomfortable and slightly clumsy for the patient over the long-term. This method of treatment is often the least expensive and requires the shortest time frame. A removable partial denture is useful in replacing the missing tooth and gum tissue. Additional teeth can be added to it in the future.

Option 4—Implant-Supported Crown

The implant-supported crown is a prosthetic replacement tooth held in place by a single implant. The advantage of this procedure is that there is no tooth preparation or shaping necessary. The areas in between the teeth are available for the patient to clean. Recent studies have shown that there is bone preservation or stabilization around the implant after it has been placed. The restoration can be designed so it is retrievable or removable by the dentist for repair or updating if necessary. The disadvantage of this procedure is that occasionally there is loosening of the screw, fracture of the restoration, and failure of the implant. In addition, the restoration does not replace the missing tissue in between teeth and occasionally the crown becomes uncemented. It should be noted, however, that clinical studies show that more than 90% of Brånemark System® implants installed more than 25 years ago are still functioning successfully today. Single teeth supported by implants have been placed since 1984, and show similar success rates.

This Is How It Works. . . .

Prior to implant placement, a treatment planning phase determines the best position of the implant and the anticipated position of the crown. This is done by a restorative dentist and a surgeon working as a team. At the first surgery, the implant is placed. A period of soft-tissue and bone healing follows. For the lower jaw, a minimum of four months of healing is required. For the upper jaw, a minimum of six months is required. Then the second surgery is performed where the implant is uncovered and the second component is placed. The purpose of this is to promote further soft-tissue healing, which takes about four weeks. Then the procedures to make the crown are performed by the restorative dentist. An impression is made and a crown is placed at the next appointment.

For some patients, when a tooth is lost, there is loss of bone and gum tissue as well. For these patients, augmentation (or building-up) of the tissue must be performed prior to implant placement. The anticipated implant sight is built up with either hard or soft material. This is done to achieve a better esthetic result or a better chance of success for the implant. This is not necessary for all implants, but many patients planning single tooth replacement with implants find that this is necessary to achieve their needs. Some augmentation procedures are relatively new and can alter the success of the implant. If successful, however, augmentation itself can make the implant option possible for patients who would otherwise not be considered implant candidates.

It is important to note that whichever treatment is selected, total success depends on a regular oral hygiene maintenance schedule with the restorative dentist or surgeon. All teeth need care, be they natural or prosthetic, and regular daily care is necessary to maintain optimal dental health.

If you have further questions concerning your options for single tooth replacement, please contact your dentist.

Information Concerning Multiple Missing Teeth

2

Patients with multiple missing teeth are faced with a number of dental issues. There is an esthetic problem, especially if the missing teeth are front teeth. And there is the functional problem of difficulty in chewing, especially if the missing teeth are back teeth, where much of food chewing occurs. The patient also risks a drifting of neighboring teeth into the space and movement of teeth in the opposite jaw.

Fortunately, there are several options available to treat multiple missing teeth. These options include a fixed partial denture, removable partial denture, and an implant-supported fixed partial denture. While some of the options are less expensive and more traditional, other, newer options may offer better long-term results. The next few paragraphs are designed to sort out the pros and cons of each treatment option for you in order to help you decide which one is right for you.

Option 1—Removable Partial Denture

A removable partial denture is a set of replacement teeth and gums made of metal and acrylic. Many patients find it has several disadvantages, among them, removability. It is often very bulky. Patients sometimes find that it makes speech difficult and sometimes alters taste. There is also a risk of tooth decay, gum tissue irritation, and bone problems where the partial rests. Finally, there is in some cases an esthetic problem because metal or wire may show when the patient smiles. It should be noted, however, that overall treatment time for this option is relatively short and cost can be relatively low. The removable partial denture effectively replaces missing teeth and gum tissue. It serves to stabilize the bite and to prevent unwanted drifting of adjacent teeth into the space.

Option 2—Fixed Partial Denture

A fixed partial denture is a prosthesis made of metal, or metal and porcelain. The neighboring teeth are trimmed down or prepared on either side of the space where teeth are missing and the partial denture is cemented over the teeth. This restoration is fixed, ie, non-removable by the patient. It can have certain problems. There is a risk of decay, nerve damage, gum tissue irritation, or bone damage. The restoration may fracture, crack, or become uncemented. A fixed partial denture replaces the missing teeth and prevents movement of neighboring teeth. This option is esthetically pleasing and functions well.

Option 3—Implant-Supported Fixed Partial Denture

In this treatment option, the prosthesis (or set of replacement teeth) is similar to the fixed partial denture described above. However, the method of installation in the patient's mouth is very different. With this option, the partial denture is held in place by implant screws which are placed in the patient's jaw bone. This method greatly reduces the risk of decay, nerve-damage, and gum tissue irritation in the jaw. Although it is fixed, it can be removed by the dentist for adjustments, repairs, or maintenance. Occasional problems can include restoration fracture and loosening or fracture of the implant screws. In a very small percentage of patients, the implants fail. This option requires two surgical procedures, described below, and a longer treatment time than some of the previously described options. It should be noted however, that clinical studies show that more than 90% of the Brånemark System® implants installed more than 25 years ago are still functioning successfully today. These implants have been used in patients with multiple missing teeth since 1967, and have a similar success rate.

This Is How It Works. . . .

For an implant-supported fixed partial denture, a cooperative treatment plan is completed by the restorative dentist and surgeon. During this period, the number and positioning of implants, and the final restorative design are planned. The first surgery follows, at which time the implants are placed. The soft tissue and the bone are then allowed to heal. In the lower jaw, a four-month healing period is necessary; in the upper jaw, a six-month period is required. During the second surgery, the implants are uncovered and a healing component is screwed into place. This component then is visible through the gum tissue. Its purpose is to promote further gum tissue healing around the implant site, a process that takes about four weeks.

Afterward, a series of appointments with the restorative dentist will include the taking of preliminary and final impressions, a metal try-in, and, finally, delivery of the restoration. For some patients, temporaries can be made during the soft-tissue healing period in order to determine the optimal esthetic shape and contour of the final fixed partial denture. This treatment time is lengthier than the others presented earlier, however, many patients now wearing implant-supported fixed partial dentures report that they are comfortable and that the replacement teeth feel and work like their own natural teeth.

After completion of the dentures, regular daily maintenance by the patient is very important. As with natural teeth, regular evaluation, maintenance and hygiene visits with your restorative dentist and/or surgeon are necessary in order to maintain optimal dental health.

If you have any questions concerning your restorative options, please contact your dentist.

Information Concerning the Edentulous Maxilla

Patients with no teeth remaining in their upper jaw face several challenges with regard to wearing a denture comfortably. Fortunately, there are now several restorative options available to help those patients. The next few pages will outline just where problems arise and the various methods available to solve those problems. This information may help you better understand your choices for successful dental treatment.

Option 1—A Complete Denture

A complete denture is a prosthesis or set of replacement teeth made of acrylic and porcelain. Its disadvantage is that being removable, it is sometimes unstable and may fall or slip out of place during speech. For some patients, there is difficulty with functioning, poor speech, poor chewing ability, and looseness of the denture, especially when natural teeth still remain in the lower jaw. As a result, some patients find that dentures need refitting from time to time. In extreme cases, dentures can fracture.

It is important to note that these problems do not occur with all denture patients. In addition, traditional dentures are less costly than other restorative methods and involve a shorter treatment time. Dental research, however, is continually working toward more predictable and comfortable replacement options. Some of the other methods are outlined below.

Option 2—Implant-Supported Overdenture

The second option for the patient with no remaining upper teeth is an implant-supported overdenture. This is a denture very similar to a conventional complete denture resting on gum tissue, except that is held in place by four or more implants in the upper jaw. This denture can be removed and reinserted by the patient. The implants are connected by a cast metal bar, which helps stabilize the implants and provides a clip or retentive mechanism to hold the denture in place. The advantage of this option is that the denture is removable and the bar and denture are accessible for daily cleaning. The implants give the denture more stability and retention, and they increase the bite force. This type of treatment allows the dentist and patient to alter profile and facial contours in order to satisfy the patient's needs. The disadvantage of this treatment option is that the implant screws can fracture or loosen, and the implants sometimes fail. The denture or the denture teeth may fracture as well. The treatment time is longer than with a conventional denture on gum tissue, and two oral surgeries are required.

This Is How It Works. . . .

A treatment planning phase is completed prior to implant placement by the restorative dentist and the oral surgeon. The number of implants, implant positioning, and final prosthesis design are determined. Implants are placed in the upper jaw at the first surgery. The upper denture is left out for a period of days to two weeks to allow the gum tissue to heal. In the upper jaw the bone must heal around the implants for six months, and then a second surgery is completed.

The surgeon uncovers the implants at the second surgery and attaches the second component which emerges through the gum tissue. The restorative dentist then begins fabrication of the overdenture and bar after a short period of soft-tissue healing. These procedures include preliminary impression, final impression, wax try-in, bar try-in, and insertion of the denture. Adjustments are made for several months after insertion of the denture.

Once all adjustments have been made to the satisfaction of both the dentist and the patient, the patient then returns for regular maintenance and reevaluation appointments.

In addition, most patients report better stability, stronger bite force, and in general, replacements that perform better.

Option 3—Implant-Supported Fixed Complete Denture

An implant-supported fixed complete denture is another option for the patient with no teeth remaining in the upper jaw. This restoration is supported by five or more implants in the upper jaw and is fixed (not removable). It is made of either (1) metal, denture acrylic, and denture teeth or (2) metal and porcelain. The advantage of this restoration is that it has better stability than a conventional, complete denture or some overdenture designs. The restoration is retrievable or removable by the dentist, but is fixed in place during patient use. This restoration has been shown to stabilize bone height over time. The disadvantage of this option is that there is occasional implant failure, screw fracture, screw loosening, or prosthesis fracture. The patient may experience occasional difficulty with daily maintenance around this fixed denture. This is due to the shape the denture takes in order to create a more esthetic result for the patient or to hide metal components. Some patients have found that there is a difficulty with speech with the fixed complete denture in the upper jaw. This is due to

2

air escape underneath the denture when some words or letters are pronounced. Many patients find that after a period of time, practice, or an adjustment, their speech returns to normal. However, in occasional cases, these speech problems continue.

This Is How It Works. . . .

The treatment planning phase is very similar to that of an implant-supported overdenture with coordinated visits by the patient to the dentist and oral surgeon for two surgical procedures and fabrication of the new teeth. The result is a prosthesis held in place by four or more implants. Again, it is removable only by a surgeon or dentist, however, this method is reported to offer maximum stability and overall performance.

It is important to note that, whichever treatment is selected, total success depends on a regular schedule of oral hygiene maintenance with the restorative dentist or surgeon. All teeth need care, be they natural or prosthetic.

If you have any questions regarding your options please contact your dentist.

Information Concerning the Edentulous Mandible

Patients with no teeth remaining in the lower jaw present a most challenging dental situation. Even with a complete lower denture, discomfort, clumsiness, and jawbone loss can continue. Dental methods have evolved, fortunately, to offer several updated options to these patients. Each option has its own set of advantages and disadvantages. The next few paragraphs are designed to inform you about each method, so that you can make an educated choice as to which treatment might work best for you.

Option 1—Complete Denture

A complete denture is a prosthesis made of acrylic and denture teeth. The advantages of this method are familiarity and cost, but the outcome can be more problematic than with other treatment choices. The denture is removable and, for some patients, this can result in sore tissue, difficult function, poor speech, and poor chewing ability. There is continued bone loss underneath the denture and many adjustments or soft-tissue conditioners are often necessary.

It is important to note that these problems do not occur with all denture patients. In addition, traditional dentures are less costly than other restorative methods and involve a shorter treatment time. Dental research, however, is continually working toward more predictable and comfortable replacement options. Some of the other methods are outlined below.

Option 2—Overdenture Supported by Implants

This is a denture very similar to a lower complete denture. The difference is that it is held in place by two or more implant screws that have been placed in the lower jawbone. The denture can be removed and reinserted by the patient. It is attached to the implants with a clip or attachment mechanism that helps hold the denture in place. The denture shape allows profile and esthetic control by the restorative dentist with the patient's input. This prosthesis results in increased bite force. There is also better retention and stability of the prosthesis with this option. Implants are placed in a very predictable region in the front part of the lower jaw for this prosthesis. Occasionally, denture repairs and replacement of clips are needed. There is also continued bone loss in the very posterior region, where the denture rests; however, this can be remedied by refitting the denture from time to time.

2

This Is How It Works....

For this procedure, a treatment planning phase is first completed by the restorative dentist and the oral surgeon. The number of implants, the implant position, and final prosthesis design is determined. Implants are placed in the anterior portion of the lower jaw at the first surgery. The lower denture is left out for several days to two weeks to allow for initial soft-tissue healing. Then the denture is replaced. The bone and soft tissues are allowed to heal for a minimum of four months and then the implants are uncovered. The surgeon uncovers the implants at the second surgery and screws components to the top of the implants. A period of soft-tissue healing follows. The restorative dentist then completes the bar and lower overdenture. The dentist makes preliminary impressions, final impressions, a bite registration, a wax try-in, and delivery of the dentures. After delivery of the dentures, a period of adjustment follows.

After completion of the dentures, regular daily maintenance by the patient is very important. As with natural teeth, regular evaluation, maintenance, and hygiene visits with the restorative dentist and/or surgeon are necessary in order to maintain the optimal dental health of the implants.

Option 3—Implant-Supported Complete Denture

If this option is selected, the patient has four to six implants placed in the lower front jaw. The advantage of this option is that it is a fixed restoration, which remains in the patient's mouth. The patient has a greater bite force and ability to chew a wider variety of foods. This option has more stability and retention than a conventional complete denture or an overdenture on implants. A disadvantage is that this procedure requires more implants. Occasionally the design of the denture makes it challenging for the patient to clean it on a daily basis. In general, this fixed denture is more difficult to clean around than the overdenture.

As with other prostheses, the fixed complete denture may break, the metal may break, screws may fracture, and screws may become loosened. However, it is important to note that this restorative option has shown, in over 25 years of clinical studies, a success rate greater than 90%. For this procedure, the treatment planning phase is the same as that outlined for the overdenture supported by implants.

It is important to note that, whichever treatment is selected, total success depends on a regular oral hygiene maintenance schedule with the restorative dentist or surgeon. All teeth need care, be they natural or prosthetic, and regular daily upkeep is necessary to maintain optimal dental health.

If you have any questions concerning your dental restorative options, please contact your dentist.

Patient Economy

Determining a reasonable fee for a restorative dental service is often a challenging undertaking. This section is intended to help the clinician establish a fee for implant restorative procedures. The clinician should note that each patient situation is unique. A more challenging situation would of course require a more significant fee. The clinician is encouraged to consider all of the procedures to be performed for the potential implant patient prior to establishing a fee.

Overall Fee Considerations for the Patient

1. Treatment planning
   a. Examination
   b. Radiographs
   c. Diagnostic casts
   d. Photos
   e. Surgical-radiographic guide
   f. Fees
      1. Some clinicians have fees for each treatment planning phase separate from the restorative phase of the implant treatment. These clinicians have found that more patients explore the implant option than actually have implants placed. Some patients go through the treatment planning phase and then stop their own treatment.
2. First surgery/implant placement
   a. This is normally a surgical responsibility and the restorative dentist is not involved.
   b. Some clinicians quote only the restorative fee and have the surgeon quote the surgical fee. The patient simply adds the two figures.
   c. Some restorative clinicians are hesitant to quote surgical fees because there are often additional surgical procedures that are necessary. These additional procedures may include pre-prosthetic surgery or augmentation procedures. The addition of these procedures to a treatment plan may significantly alter the patient's total fee.
3. Postsurgical care
   a. Adjustment after first surgery and relining of existing denture (tissue treatment)
      1. This procedure is often performed by the restorative dentist.

   2. The restorative dentist should attempt to predict the interval and frequency of appointments at the beginning of treatment as this will affect the amount of time and materials spent on this procedure. This will in turn affect the total fee for the patient.
   3. Fee determination options:
      a. Fee per visit based on length of appointment and materials used;
      b. Estimated fee for tissue treatment included in total for prosthesis.
   b. Transitional prosthesis
      1. Some patients may require the fabrication of a transitional or interim prosthesis that is worn during the period of healing after the surgeries.
      2. This prosthesis may be a complete denture, a removable-treatment partial denture, or a fixed provisional restoration.
      3. The restorative clinician is encouraged to compensate for this procedure in the total estimated patient fee.
4. Second surgery—implants uncovered
   a. Healing abutment placement
      1. This procedure is usually performed by the surgeon.
   b. Definitive abutment selection and connection (two options)
      1. Placement by the surgeon after joint restorative-surgical consultation
         a. The advocates of this technique suggest that the surgeon can best confirm that the abutment is seated because the surgeon has the second-phase surgical instrumentation. This equipment allows the surgeon to remove any hard or soft tissue that may be preventing the complete seating of the abutment.

3

b. The surgeon often takes responsibility for seating the abutment because the restorative dentist does not have the torque-controller instrumentation. The surgeon can assure that the abutment is seated and that the screw joint is closed for a predictable torsional load.

2. Placement by the restorative dentist

a. Some clinicians feel that the person who is going to restore the patient should select the abutment and place it.

b. This is advocated because some dentists have had problems with placing abutments and then having to change them because of unacceptable heights or position.

3. Protocol

a. Each team of restorative dentists and surgeons will determine its own protocol for abutment placement. The person placing the abutment may vary depending on the clinical situation. It is important prior to implant placement to determine who will place the abutment so it may be added to that clinician's total estimated fee. If this is not done, either the patient is surprised with an additional fee or the clinician has increased cost without a patient fee to compensate.

c. Provisional prosthesis after second surgery

1. Adjustment of removable prosthesis

a. For many patients, adjusting the removable prosthesis and placing a tissue conditioner is necessary.

b. This tissue-treatment material must be changed at intervals during the healing after the second surgery and while the prosthesis is being fabricated. Compensation for this service should be included in the total estimated restorative fee.

2. Fixed provisional restorations on implants

a. Some patients will have a provisional restoration fabricated. This restoration will often require two clinical appointments, implant components, and a laboratory fee. The clinician should take this procedure into account when estimating the restorative fee.

5. Prosthesis fabrication procedures fee

a. The procedures necessary to fabricate the prosthesis are what most clinicians consider when establishing an estimated restorative fee. It is obvious from the preceding discussion that the procedures involved in fabricating the prosthesis are only a portion of the total service provided for the patient.

b. Fee determination for prosthesis fabrication is based on the following

1. Clinical procedures and time

2. Laboratory fee

3. Restorative component cost

4. Adjustments (especially for removable prostheses)

a. At the beginning of treatment, some clinicians will include a limitation on the number of adjustments after delivery of the restoration.

b. Other clinicians will limit the time during which adjustments will be included in the initial restorative fee (eg, two months after delivery).

c. After these limitations, some offices charge an additional fee based on clinical time spent and materials used.

d. Of course, some flexibility is necessary.

6. Maintenance fees

   a. Patients should be informed that maintenance and re-evaluation fees are separate from the restorative fee. This concept may be new for completely edentulous patients who often disappear from practices for years.

   b. Maintenance fees may include, but are not limited to, the following:

      1. Prophylaxis, radiographs, and examination

      2. Overdenture soft-tissue conditioners or clip replacement

      3. Tooth replacement after several years (for some completely edentulous patients with fixed prosthesis)

      4. Screw tightening or replacement

   c. Repair policy:

      1. Each office is encouraged to establish a repair and replacement policy.

      2. Some clinicians offer a guarantee or warranty for the prosthesis. This also serves as a marketing aid for the implant portion of their practice.

      3. Other clinicians have a repair policy, but it is not emphasized in the patient presentation.

Fee Determination Exercise

This exercise is intended to help the clinician determine a reasonable fee for a procedure in a particular practice. The intention is to determine how much money the practice must take in, per hour, in order to cover overhead expenses and provide a particular net-income goal. The numbers used in this example are fictitious and are not intended as suggestions for hourly fees or goals. Each practice is unique and should perform its own calculations based on existing overhead expense and net-income goal.

Private Practice Evaluation	**Example**
Total monthly expense (overhead)	$16,000
Number of days worked per month	20
Number of hours worked per day	8
Number of hours worked per month	160
Expense per hour	$100
Yearly net-income goal	$192,000
Monthly net-income goal	$16,000
Number of days worked per month	20
Number of hours worked per day	8
Number of hours worked per month	160
Net-income goal per hour	$100
Receipts goal per hour	$200

This information can be used to help determine the restorative fees for osseointegrated implants.

Procedure Overview and Clinical Time Determination

In this section, options for restorative treatments have been divided into four types:

1. **Single Missing Tooth**
2. **Partially Edentulous—Fixed Partial Denture**
3. **Completely Edentulous—Fixed, Detachable Prosthesis**
4. **Overdenture, Implant-Supported**

This is intended to assist the clinician with a reasonable fee determination:

- The clinician may estimate the hours required for a procedure as a basis for determining the estimated clinical fee.
- The estimated hours are multiplied by the practice's hourly-receipts goal to determine the fee.

Total hours × Receipts goal per hour = Estimated clinical fees

Single Tooth Replacement

Patient _____ Date _____

Procedure	Time (Hours)	Fee ($)
1. Treatment planning		
• Clinical examination	_____	_____
• Mounted diagnostic casts	_____	_____
• Diagnostic wax-up	_____	_____
• Radiographs	_____	_____
• Surgical guide	_____	_____
• Fabrication of provisional prosthesis	_____	_____
• Try-in of diagnostic wax-up	_____	_____
2. First surgery: implant placed	_____	_____
3. Provisional prosthesis adjustment (minimum: maxilla—6 months, mandible—4 months)	_____	_____
4. Second surgery: implant uncovered and healing abutment placed	_____	_____
5. Provisional adjustment during soft-tissue healing	_____	_____
6. Definitive abutment placed (by surgeon or restorative dentist)	_____	_____
7. Restorative appointments		
• Fixed provisional	_____	_____
• Final impression	_____	_____
• Cementation	_____	_____
• Re-evaluation	_____	_____
8. Subtotals (clinical time and clinical fee)	_____	_____
9. Laboratory fee		
• Components	_____	_____
• Metal	_____	_____
• Labor	_____	_____
Total restorative fee:	_____	_____

Many clinicians add the laboratory fee (because it is often significant for this procedure) to the clinical fee to arrive at the total restorative fee for a single tooth replacement.

Partially Edentulous—Fixed Partial Denture

Patient _____ Date _____

Procedure	Time (Hrs)	Fee ($)
1. Treatment planning		
• Clinical examination	____	____
• Mounted diagnostic casts	____	____
• Diagnostic wax-up	____	____
• Radiographs	____	____
• Surgical guide	____	____
• Fabrication of provisional prosthesis	____	____
• Try-in of diagnostic wax-up	____	____
2. First surgery: implant placed	____	____
3. Provisional prosthesis adjustment (minimum: maxilla—6 months, mandible—4 months)	____	____
4. Second surgery: implant uncovered and healing abutment placed	____	____
5. Provisional prosthesis adjustment during soft-tissue healing	____	____
6. Definitive abutment placed (by surgeon or restorative dentist)	____	____

Procedure	Time (Hrs)	Fee ($)
7. Provisional prosthesis options:		
• Soft-tissue conditioner for treatment partial denture	____	____
• Fixed, screw-retained provisional prosthesis (laboratory processed)	____	____
8. Restorative procedures		
• Initial impression (optional)	____	____
• Final impressions	____	____
• Maxillo-mandibular registration	____	____
• Metal framework try-in	____	____
• Placement of restoration	____	____
• Re-evaluation	____	____
9. Subtotals (clinical time and clinical fee)	____	____
10. Laboratory fee		
• Components	____	____
• Metal	____	____
• Labor	____	____
Total restorative fee:	____	____

Many clinicians add the laboratory fee (often significant) to the estimated clinical fee to determine the restorative fee for the partially edentulous implant patient. Some use a formula to determine the fee per unit.

Completely Edentulous—Fixed Detachable Prosthesis

Patient _____ Date _____

Procedure	Time (Hrs)	Fee ($)
1. Treatment planning		
• Clinical examination	____	____
• Mounted diagnostic casts	____	____
• Diagnostic wax-up	____	____
• Radiographs	____	____
• Surgical guides	____	____
• Fabrication of provisional prosthesis	____	____
• Try-in of diagnostic wax-up	____	____
2. First surgery: implant placed	____	____
3. Provisional prosthesis adjustment (minimum: maxilla—6 months, mandible—4 months)	____	____
4. Second surgery: implant uncovered and healing abutment placed	____	____
5. Adjustment complete denture (soft-tissue healing)	____	____
6. Third surgery (optional). Definitive abutments are placed if not done at second surgery	____	____

Procedure	Time (Hrs)	Fee ($)
7. Restorative procedures		
• Initial impression (optional)	____	____
• Final impressions	____	____
• Maxillo-mandibular registration	____	____
• Wax trial denture	____	____
• Framework try-in	____	____
• Second framework try-in (optional)	____	____
• Second wax try-in on metal framework (optional)	____	____
• Placement of restoration	____	____
• Re-evaluation	____	____
8. Subtotals (clinical time and restorative fee)	____	____
9. Laboratory fee		
• Components	____	____
• Metal	____	____
• Labor	____	____
Total restorative fee:	____	____

Some clinicians add the laboratory cost to the estimated clinical fee to calculate the total restorative fee. Some multiply the number of teeth in the prosthesis by the fee for a single unit of fixed prosthodontics on a natural tooth.

Overdenture

Patient _____ Date _____

Procedure	Time (Hrs)	Fee ($)
1. Treatment planning		
• Clinical examination	____	____
• Mounted diagnostic casts	____	____
• Diagnostic wax-up	____	____
• Radiographs	____	____
• Surgical guides	____	____
• Fabrication of provisional prosthesis	____	____
• Try-in of diagnostic wax-up	____	____
2. First surgery: implant placed	____	____
3. Adjustment of complete denture (minimum: 6 months, maxilla; 4 months, mandible)	____	____
4. Second surgery: implant uncovered and healing or definitive abutment placed	____	____
5. Adjustment of complete denture (soft-tissue healing)	____	____
6. Third surgery (optional). Placement of definitive abutment if not done prior to this appointment	____	____

Procedure	Time (Hrs)	Fee ($)
7. Restorative appointments		
a. Option 1		
• Initial impression	____	____
• Final impression	____	____
• Maxillo-mandibular registration	____	____
• Wax trial denture	____	____
• Bar try-in (section)	____	____
• (Try-in of soldered bar)	____	____
• Placement of restoration	____	____
• Adjustments and re-evaluation	____	____
b. Option 2		
• Initial impression	____	____
• Bar try-in and final impression	____	____
• Maxillo-mandibular relations	____	____
• Wax trial denture	____	____
• Placement of prosthesis	____	____
• Adjustments and re-evaluation	____	____
8. Subtotals (clinical time and fee)	____	____
9. Laboratory fee		
• Labor	____	____
• Metal	____	____
• Component fee	____	____
Total restorative fee:	____	____

Other Considerations

▼ Additional Fees

1. Treatment planning phase
2. Prosthesis adjustment
3. Provisional restorations
4. Maintenance and recall appointments
5. Transitional prosthesis

▼ Insurance Coverage

1. Insurance codes

American Dental Association. CDT-2: Current Dental Terminology, ed 2. Chicago: American Dental Association, 1994:27–28.

- 0600-06199 Implant Services: "Prosthetic devices should be reported using existing fixed or removable prosthetic codes. If fixed partial denture work is performed, the crown over the implant is considered the abutment."
- 06055 "Implant connecting bar—A device attached to transmucosal abutments to stabilize and anchor a removable overdenture prosthesis . . ."
- 06080 "Implant maintenance procedures, includes: removal of prosthesis, cleansing of prosthesis and abutment and reinsertion of prosthesis."
- 06199 Unspecified implant procedure, by report: "Use for procedure which is not adequately described by code. Describe procedure."

2. Insurance coverage for implant prosthesis is inconsistent.

3

Component Costs

This clinician should attempt to predict the component cost prior to implant placement. Once this exercise is done for a specific implant and type of restoration, the information can be utilized for future patients. For instance, the clinician should know the cost of components per implant for a particular abutment and a particular clinical situation.

Patient _____ Date _____

Surgical Components

Implant   _____
Cover screw   _____
Drills   _____
Total   _____

The component cost for surgical placement of the implant is $ _____

Abutment Connection Components

Healing abutment   _____
Abutment   _____
Abutment screw   _____
Healing cap   _____
Total   _____

The component cost for abutment connection per implant is $ _____

Restorative Components (multiple implants)

Impression coping   _____
Guide pin   _____
Abutment replica   _____
Gold cylinder   _____
Gold screw   _____
Total   _____

The restorative component cost per implant is $ _____

3

Restorative Components (single tooth)

Impression coping   _____
Guide pin   _____
Implant replica   _____
Gold cylinder   _____
Ceramic cap   _____
Total   _____

The restorative component cost per implant for a single
tooth restoration is $ _____

Restorative Components—Overdenture (bar and clip)

Impression coping   _____
Guide pin   _____
Abutment replica   _____
Gold bar   _____
Gold cylinder   _____
Gold screw   _____
Clip   _____
Attachment   _____
Total   _____

The restorative component cost per implant for an overdenture retained with a bar
and clip (**not** including the cost of the plastic bar and clip) is $ _____

Restorative Components—Overdenture (ball attachment)

O-ring   _____
Ball attachment replica   _____
Spacer   _____
Total   _____

The restorative component cost per implant for an overdenture
ball attachment is $ _____

Treatment Planning Overview

▼ Initial Patient Interview

1. Chief complaint
   a. Often the patient's chief complaint about the existing prosthesis will alter the surgical and restorative procedures performed.
   b. A completely edentulous patient who dislikes the removable aspect of the existing prosthesis often requires a fixed implant restoration. Additional osseointegrated implants or surgical procedures may be necessary to accomplish this.
   c. A completely edentulous patient who complains of the mobility of the existing restoration may require a fixed or a removable prosthesis.

2. The patient's needs or goals should be recorded.
   a. It is important to note this information so that a treatment plan can be formulated in the attempt to fulfill the patient's needs.
   b. The clinician should remember that some patient goals may be unrealistic or unattainable. The patient should be notified of the limitations prior to initiating treatment so the patient can make an educated decision.

▼ Medical History Review— Screens For:

1. Mental disorder
2. Pregnancy
3. Prior radiation treatment
4. Inability to have elective surgery
5. Steroid use
6. Diabetes
7. Immune deficiency
   a. Systemic lupus erythematosis
   b. Discoid lupus erythematosis

▼ Extraoral Examination

1. Skin
2. Lips
3. TMJ
4. Muscles of mastication, facial expression
5. Profile
6. High smile line (with and without prosthesis)
   a. Record the distance from the high smile line of the lip to the residual ridge.
   b. If the residual ridge is visible, record the number of millimeters visible.
7. Low smile line (with and without prosthesis)
   a. Record the distance from the lower lip to the residual ridge.
   b. If the residual ridge is visible, record the number of millimeters visible.
   c. In the mandibular anterior region, some patients require height reduction of the alveolar ridge prior to implant placement to improve esthetics.

▼ Intraoral Examination

1. Soft tissue
   a. Buccal mucosa
   b. Vestibules
   c. Hard palate
   d. Soft palate
   e. Floor of mouth
   f. Frenum attachments
2. Teeth
   a. Restorations
   b. Caries
   c. Missing teeth
   d. Prognosis
3. Periodontal
   a. Probing depths
   b. Mobility of teeth
   c. Furcations
   d. Bleeding
   e. Crown-to-root ratio
   f. Prognosis
   g. Oral hygiene evaluation
4. Occlusal analysis
   a. Centric contact: prematurity or slide
   b. Contacts in laterotrusion and protrusion
   c. Skeletal class I, II, III
   d. Occlusal wear, facets
   e. Range of motion
   f. Plane of occlusion

▼ Radiographs

1. Full-mouth periapical radiographs
   a. Advantages
      1. Useful in analyzing remaining natural teeth
      2. Periodontal bone level can be analyzed
      3. Pathology can be identified
   b. Disadvantages
      1. Unable to view entire anatomy
2. Panoramic radiograph
   a. Advantages
      1. Low cost
      2. Full arch anatomy
      3. Low radiation exposure
   b. Disadvantages
      1. Distance measurement less precise than other methods
      2. Overlap
      3. Distortion
      4. Magnification
3. Tomogram
   a. Advantages
      1. Low to moderate radiation exposure
      2. Moderate cost
      3. Cross-section view
      4. Direct measurement on film
   b. Disadvantages
      1. Lack of detail in some views
4. Computerized tomogram
   a. Advantages
      1. Good detail
      2. Cross-section view
      3. Direct measurement on film
      4. Most predictable measurements
   b. Disadvantages
      1. High cost
      2. Higher radiation exposure

▼ Mounted Diagnostic Casts

1. Vertical space available
2. Mesiodistal space available
3. Ridge width
4. Maxillo-mandibular relations: class I, II, III skeletal
5. Anatomical structures
   a. Palatal tori
   b. Tuberosities
   c. Lingual tori
   d. Bony exostosis

▼ Diagnostic Wax-up

1. Denture teeth useful
2. Used to fabricate surgical guide

▼ Photographs

1. Pretreatment

▼ Consultation

1. Oral surgeon
2. Periodontist
3. Endodontist
4. Orthodontist
5. Laboratory technician

4

▼ Surgical Guide

1. Purpose
   a. The purpose of the surgical guide is to communicate to the surgeon the ideal position of the planned prosthetic teeth.
   b. The surgeon uses this information to place the implant in appropriate position so that it can be restored optimally.

2. Completely edentulous procedure
   a. Duplicate existing complete denture if esthetics, occlusion, and distance between arches are adequate.
   b. If the complete denture is inadequate or there is none, fabricate one to the wax trial denture appointment and duplicate.

3. Partially edentulous procedures (2 options)
   a. Make an impression of diagnostic wax-up and pour in autopolymerized clear acrylic resin. Contour segment and index to incisal edges.
   b. Make an impression of diagnostic wax-up and pour in stone. Fabricate a 2-mm vacuum-formed index of cast. Trim and prepare for surgery.

4. Use as a joint surgical-radiographic guide
   a. The guide can be worn by the patient during the radiographic procedure.
   b. Metal markers or gutta percha can be placed in the guide for periapical, panoramic, or tomographic radiographs.
   c. For computerized axial tomograms, the guide can be coated with a radiopaque material such as barium sulfate.
   d. Metal must be excluded with computerized axial tomography to prevent backscatter.
   e. Guide may be used at the surgical augmentation of the ridge. The surgeon can predict how much the ridge must be augmented by using the guide and noting the position of the buccal surface and free gingival margin.
   f. For the partially edentulous patient, the guide should communicate the position of the incisal edge, free gingival margin, and labial surface of the planned prosthetic tooth.

▼ Team Approach

It is critical for the restorative dentist, laboratory technician, and surgeon to communicate in detail prior to implant placement. This will reduce the interesting moments in the restoration of the patient and assure a more predictable esthetic result.

Diagnosis and Treatment Planning Flow Sheets

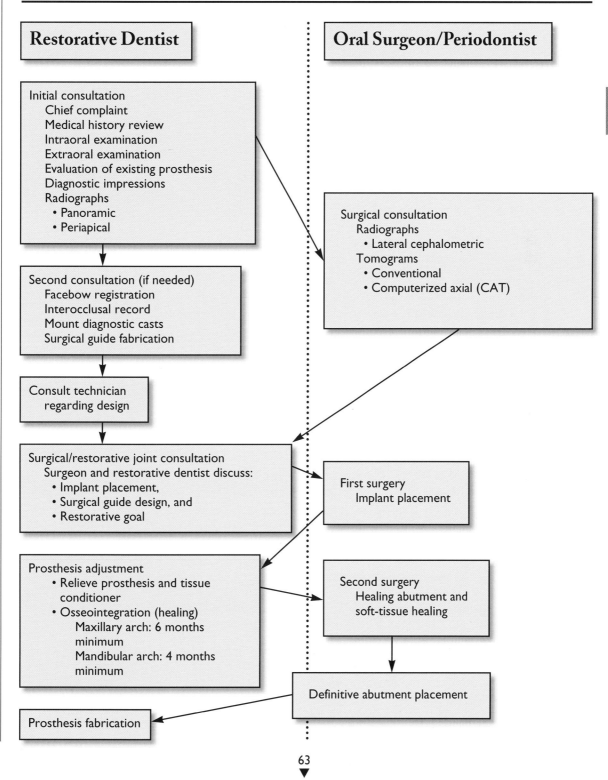

Restorative Dentist

Oral Surgeon/Periodontist

4

Initial consultation
    Chief complaint
    Medical history review
    Intraoral examination
    Extraoral examination
    Evaluation of existing prosthesis
    Diagnostic impressions
    Radiographs
    • Panoramic
    • Periapical

Surgical consultation
    Radiographs
    • Lateral cephalometric
    Tomograms
    • Conventional
    • Computerized axial (CAT)

Second consultation (if needed)
    Facebow registration
    Interocclusal record
    Mount diagnostic casts
    Surgical guide fabrication

Consult technician
    regarding design

Surgical/restorative joint consultation
    Surgeon and restorative dentist discuss:
    • Implant placement,
    • Surgical guide design, and
    • Restorative goal

First surgery
    Implant placement

Prosthesis adjustment
    • Relieve prosthesis and tissue
        conditioner
    • Osseointegration (healing)
        Maxillary arch: 6 months
        minimum
        Mandibular arch: 4 months
        minimum

Second surgery
    Healing abutment and
    soft-tissue healing

Definitive abutment placement

Prosthesis fabrication

Treatment Planning Forms

Included in this section are sample forms to assist the dental implant team in providing optimal patient care.

- The treatment planning checklist is intended to be utilized by the restorative dentist to assure that all presurgical information is collected.

- The surgical referral form is intended to be filled out by the restorative dentist and sent to the surgeon. After evaluation, the surgeon may fill out the surgical recommendations and any additional diagnostic information needed from the restorative dentist.

- The laboratory consultation form may be sent by the restorative dentist with diagnostic casts to the laboratory technician. The technician can often provide treatment or design suggestions to facilitate a more predictable restoration. The technician may also provide the restorative dentist with a laboratory fee estimate and suggest other diagnostic information needed prior to implant placement.

Treatment Planning Checklist

Patient: _____   Date_____

_____ **Patient Interview**
Chief complaint _____
Need_____
_____ **Medical History** _____
_____ **Extraoral Exam** _____
    _____ High smile (maxilla)_____
    _____ Low smile (mandible) _____
_____ **Intraoral Exam**

_____

_____ **Radiographs**
    _____ Full mouth periapicals
    _____ Panoramic radiograph
    _____ Tomograms
    _____ Computerized axial tomogram
    _____ Lateral cephalometric
_____ **Mounted Diagnostic Casts**
_____ **Diagnostic Wax-up**
_____ **Photographs**
_____ **Consultation**
    _____ Oral Surgeon_____
    _____ Periodontist_____
    _____ Endodontist_____
    _____ Orthodontist_____
    _____ Laboratory Technician _____
_____ **Guide: Radiographic** _____ **Surgical** _____

Considerations:

_____

_____

Proposed Treatment Plan:

_____

_____

_____

Treatment Planning: Surgical Referral Form

Patient Name:_____

Restorative Doctor:_____

Restorative Recommendations: _____
_____
_____

Date Completed: **Comments:**

_____   Patient's need _____ Fixed _____Removable _____

_____   Medical history_____

_____   Extraoral exam_____

_____   Intraoral exam _____

_____   Mounted diagnostic casts_____

_____   Diagnostic wax-up _____

_____   Photographs _____

_____   Radiographs _____ fmx _____ pan _____ tomo _____ ct _____lat ceph

_____   Surgical Guide _____

Diagnosis:

Maxilla _____

Mandible _____

Prognosis of Existing Teeth:

Good prognosis—teeth #s _____

Guarded prognosis—teeth #s _____

Poor prognosis—teeth #s_____

Treatment Plan (proposed):

Maxilla _____

Mandible _____

Proposed Prosthesis Design:

Maxilla   **Mandible**

Surgical Recommendations: _____
_____
_____

Suggest: **Surgeon:**_____

_____   Mounted diagnostic casts _____

_____   Surgical guide (type): _____

_____   Radiographs: _____ fmx _____ pan _____ tomo _____ ct _____lat ceph

Treatment Planning: Laboratory Consultation Form

Patient: _____   **Doctor:** _____

Date: _____

Patient Objective _____ Fixed _____ Removable

Proposed Treatment Plan:

_____

_____

Proposed Prosthesis Design:

Maxilla   **Mandible**

_____   _____

_____   _____

_____   _____

_____   _____

_____   _____

Proposed Materials:
  1. Porcelain-fused-to-metal _____
  2. Acrylic-to-metal _____
  3. Occlusal materials: gold _____ acrylic _____ porcelain _____

Proposed Components:
  1. Abutments _____
     _____

Laboratory—Estimated Costs:
  1. Component _____
  2. Laboratory labor _____
  3. Metal cost_____

Total Estimated Cost: _____

Information Needed:

_____ Mounted diagnostic casts   _____ Presurgical diagnostic wax-up

_____ Surgical-radiographic guide   _____ Diagnostic wax-up

Further Treatment or Design Suggestions: _____

_____

_____

_____

Treatment Planning and Decision Making

This section includes a series of forms and patient examples that may be useful in treatment planning and decision making. On a daily basis, the restorative dentist evaluates dental problems and automatically formulates a treatment plan. The restoration of osseointegrated implants requires the same thought process but sometimes the treatment is more elaborate or lengthy. The dentist first analyzes and lists the problems the patient presents. This problem list is used to justify the proposed treatment plan and alternatives. The patient is presented with the treatment plan, alternatives, and the advantages and disadvantages of each option. Then the patient selects a treatment plan with the guidance of the dentist. After the definitive treatment plan is determined, the treatment sequence is planned.

▼ Problem List Form

The problem list form is used in an attempt to create a rationale for proposed treatment. Problem types are listed under the regions of the mouth were they occur, and potential problem areas are listed under the procedures used to test them. Some of the categories considered include:

1. Teeth
   a. Numbers
   b Existing conditions: restorations; chipped, fractured teeth
   c. Vitality of teeth
   d. Caries

2. Periodontium
   a. Crown/root ratio
   b. Bone support
   c. Mobility
   d. Furcations
   e. Pocket depths
   f. Mucogingival problems (inadequate keratinized attached gingiva)

3. Radiographic analysis
   a. Periapical pathology
   b. Vertical bone height in edentulous region
   c. Radiopaque regions or objects
   d. Radiolucent regions

4. Esthetic analysis
   a. High smile line—maxillary arch
   b. Ridge defect from previous extractions
   c. Extraction sites and ridge contour
   d. Low smile line—mandibular arch

5. Occlusal analysis

6. Diagnostic casts
   a. Vertical space available for prosthesis
   b. Ridge width
   c. Maxillo-mandibular relations

▼ Treatment Plan Form

This form lists the proposed dental care and alternatives.

1. List teeth, areas, and proposed treatments.
2. Consider the advantages and disadvantages of proposed treatment as discussed in Chapter 1.
3. Consider the alternatives and their advantages and disadvantages.
4. Consider:
   a. Longevity of existing restorations
   b. Prognosis of remaining natural teeth
   c. Improvement of function
   d. Improvement of esthetics

5. Determine the *convertibility* of your proposed treatment plan. If other teeth or restorations fail, how easily can the patient be returned to optimal dental health?

6. If few teeth remain, will they compromise the maintenance or long-term success of the prosthesis? Sometimes a simpler, more predictable prosthetic solution can be achieved by removal of the few remaining teeth.

7. Prior to treatment, can the prognosis of the proposed treatment plan be improved with:

   a. Orthodontic therapy

   b. Pre-prosthetic surgery

     1. Extractions

     2. Ridge contouring

     3. Removal of tori or exostosis

     4. Tuberosity reduction

     5. Osteotomy

     6. Bone augmentation

     7. Soft tissue augmentation

   c. Periodontic therapy

   d. Endodontic therapy

▼ Treatment Sequence Form

At the beginning of treatment, the restorative dentist should determine the sequence of treatment to be followed. This form can be used to list all of the procedures in order of planned completion. Specialist referral can also be included in order to track the patient's progress during treatment.

1. List procedures and appointments in sequential order.

2. Include referrals and procedures to be performed by specialist.

3. Use list or flow-sheet format.

▼ Sample Forms

Several illustrated patient examples are included:

- The completely edentulous patient
- A partially edentulous patient who must become edentulous and then have implants placed

PROBLEM LIST

Patient **Number One**   Doctor _____

Date	Problem	Prognosis	Treatment
	MAXILLARY COMPLETE DENTURE		COMPLETE DENTURE
	LOOSE	GOOD	
	MANDIBULAR COMPLETE DENTURE		IMPLANTS
	SORENESS, LOOSE, NO RIDGE	POOR	FIXED PROSTHESIS

5

TREATMENT PLAN

Patient _____ **Number One** _____ **Doctor** _____

Location Tooth or Arch #	Treatment	Fee	Alternative	Fee	Completion Date
MAXILLA	COMPLETE DENTURE				
MANDIBLE	FIXED DETACHABLE		COMPLETE DENTURE		
	PROSTHESIS				

TREATMENT SEQUENCING WORKSHEET

Patient _____ **Number One** _____   **Doctor** _____

RESTORATIVE DENTIST	PERIODONTIST/ORAL SURGEON
TREATMENT PLANNING	
	SURGICAL CONSULT
INTERIM DENTURES (IF EXISTING INADEQUATE)	RADIOGRAPHS
SURGICAL GUIDE (DUPLICATE DENTURE)	
	FIRST STAGE
	IMPLANTS PLACED
ADJUST & SOFT LINE DENTURE	
HEALING (OSSEOINTEGRATION)	
4 MONTHS MIN. MANDIBLE,	
6 MONTHS MIN. MAXILLA	
	SECOND STAGE
	IMPLANTS UNCOVERED
SOFT-TISSUE HEALING	
DEFINITIVE ABUTMENT PLACEMENT	
INITIAL IMPRESSION	
FINAL IMPRESSION	
RECORDS	
WAX TRY-IN	
METAL FRAMEWORK TRY-IN	
DELIVERY OF MAXILLARY COMPLETE	
DENTURE & MANDIBULAR FIXED PROSTHESIS	
1 WEEK RE-EVALUATION	
RECALL & MAINTENANCE	

PROBLEM LIST

Patient _____ **Number Two** _____   **Doctor** _____

Date	Problem	Prognosis	Treatment
	1) MISSING		
	2) 3 : 1 CR/ROOT PERIAPICAL	POOR	EXTRACTION
	3) M CARIES, 5; 1 CR/ROOT	POOR	EXTRACTION
	4) 2 : 1 CR/ROOT RATION, MD	POOR	EXTRACTION
	5) M CARIES; 2 : 1 CR/ROOT RATIO	POOR	EXTRACTION
	6) 3 : 1 CR/ROOT RATIO	POOR	EXTRACTION
	7) 6 : 1 CR/ROOT RATIO	POOR	EXTRACTION
	8) 3 : 1 CR/ROOT RATIO	POOR	EXTRACTION
	9) 3 : 1 CR/ROOT RATIO	POOR	EXTRACTION
	10) 5 : 1 CR/ROOT RATIO	POOR	EXTRACTION
	11) 1 : 1 CR/ROOT RATIO	GOOD	(EXTRACTION)
	12) 2 : 1 CR/ROOT RATIO	POOR	(EXTRACTION)
	13) 1 : 1 CR/ROOT RATIO	GOOD	(EXTRACTION)
	14) 6 : 1 CR/ROOT RATIO	POOR	EXTRACTION
	15) 6 : 1 CR/ROOT RATIO	POOR	EXTRACTION
	16) MISSING		
	17) MISSING		
	18) MISSING		
	19) MISSING		
	20) MISSING		
	21) 3 : 1 CR/ROOT RATIO	POOR	EXTRACTION
	22) MD CARIES, PA RADIOLUC. 4 : 1	POOR	EXTRACTION
	23) 2 : 1 CR/ROOT RATIO	FAIR	EXTRACTION
	24) 2 : 1 CR/ROOT RATIO	FAIR	EXTRACTION
	25) MISSING		
	26) 2 : 1 CR/ROOT RATIO	FAIR	EXTRACTION
	27) 4 : 1 CR/ROOT RATIO	POOR	EXTRACTION
	28) 3 : 1 CR/ROOT RATIO	POOR	EXTRACTION
	29) 3 : 1 CR/ROOT RATIO	POOR	EXTRACTION
	30) MISSING		
	31) MISSING		
	32) MISSING		
			A. MAX. IMMED. COMP.
			B. MAND. IMMED. COMP.
			C. MAX. COMP. DENT.
			D. MAND. FIXED DETACH.

TREATMENT PLAN

Patient _____ **Number Two** _____ **Doctor** _____

Location Tooth or Arch #	Treatment	Fee	Alternative	Fee	Completion Date
2-16	EXTRACTION				
MAXILLARY	IMMEDIATE				
	DENTURE				
MAXILLARY	COMPLETE DENTURE		MAXILLARY RELINE		
21-29	EXTRACTION				
MANDIBULAR	IMMEDIATE				
	DENTURE				
MANDIBULAR	FIXED DETACHABLE		1. OVERDENTURE-		
	PROSTHESIS		IMPLANT		
			2. COMPLETE		
			DENTURE		
			3. MANDIBULAR		
			RELINE		

TREATMENT SEQUENCING WORKSHEET

Patient Number Two   **Doctor** _____

RESTORATIVE DENTIST	PERIODONTIST/ORAL SURGEON
DIAGNOSIS AND TREATMENT PLANNING	
↓	
1° IMPRESSIONS	
FINAL IMPRESSIONS	
MAXILLO-MANDIBULAR RECORDS	
	EXTRACTION OF TEETH
INSERTION OF MAXILLARY &	
MANDIBULAR IMMEDIATE COMPLETE DENTURE	
↓	
HEALING/TISSUE TREATMENT	
	SURGICAL RE-EVALUATION
	RADIOGRAPHS
FABRICATION OF IMPLANT PLACEMENT GUIDE	
(DUPLICATE MANDIBULAR DENTURE)	
	FIRST STAGE
	PLACEMENT OF OSSEOINTEGRATED
	IMPLANTS (MANDIBLE)
SOFT LINE MANDIBULAR DENTURE	
↓	
HEALING OSSEOINTEGRATION	
(MIN. 4 MOS MANDIBLE, 6 MOS. MAXILLA)	SECOND STAGE SURGERY
	IMPLANTS UNCOVERED
	DEFINITIVE ABUTMENTS
SOFT-TISSUE HEALING	
INITIAL IMPRESSION (MAX. & MAND.)	
FINAL IMPRESSION (MAX. & MAND.)	
RECORDS	
WAX TRY-IN	
METAL FRAMEWORK TRY-IN	
DELIVERY OF MAXILLARY COMPLETE DENTURE	
& MANDIBULAR FIXED DETACHABLE PROSTHESIS	
↓	
ONE WEEK RE-EVALUATION	
↓	
RECALL & MAINTENANCE	

PROBLEM LIST

Patient _____   **Doctor** _____

Date	Problem	Prognosis	Treatment

5

TREATMENT PLAN

Patient _____   **Doctor** _____

Location Tooth or Arch #	Treatment	Fee	Alternative	Fee	Completion Date

TREATMENT SEQUENCING WORKSHEET

Patient _____   **Doctor** _____

Single Missing Tooth

Presurgical Needs

1. Full-mouth periapical radiographs
2. Panoramic radiograph
3. Tomogram (in special instances)
4. Mounted diagnostic casts
5. Periodontal examination and charting
6. Guide: surgical/radiographic

Considerations

1. Situations in which implant-supported single-tooth restorations are avoided by some clinicians
   a. Deep vertical overlap occlusion
   b. Cuspids
   c. First molars
   d. Mandibular incisors width (because of the narrow mesiodistal width of the edentulous space)
2. Relative contraindications[1]
   a. Unrealistic expectations
   b. Bruxism
   c. Epilepsy

3. Space requirements[1,2]
   a. Goal
      1. The goal is to place the implant in the edentulous space and avoid damaging the neighboring structures.
      2. The surgeon should identify and avoid the adjacent tooth and periodontal ligament.
      3. Attention should be paid to the position, size, and shape of the interdental papilla.
      4. Careful surgical technique should be followed to preserve the interdental papilla.
   b. Mesiodistal width (Fig 6–1)

implant	=	4 mm
bone ea. side	=	1 mm + 1 mm
periodontal lig.	=	.25 + .25 mm
Total needed	=	6.5 – 7.0 mm

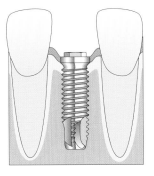

Fig 6-1

   c. Buccolingual width

      The implant must be surrounded by bone; assume the goal is 1 mm of bone surrounding all aspects of implant. For a 4-mm implant, you need 6 mm width. For a 5-mm implant, 7 mm of buccolingual space is needed. (Fig 6–2)

      Evaluate width using:

      1. Diagnostic cast measurement
      2. Ridge mapping with caliper and anesthetic
         a. If ridge is inadequate at surgery, consider augmentation.
      3. Computerized axial tomogram
      4. Tomogram
   d. Orthodontics

      If inadequate space exists the clinician should always remember that orthodontics may be useful.

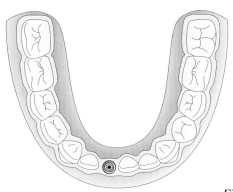

Fig 6-2

e. Vertical space[3]
1. Available vertical space (ie, from the crest of the residual alveolar bone to the opposing dentition) should be evaluated by the clinician prior to surgery, intraorally or on diagnostic casts. Soft-tissue thickness is estimated (maxillary, 2 mm; mandibular, 1 mm). If the actual thickness is greater, the clinician will have more vertical space than anticipated.

2. Required vertical space for internal hexagonal EsthetiCone gold cylinder is 6.7 mm from the superior aspect of implant to opposing occlusion. (Fig 6-3)

3. Required vertical space for CeraOne: (Fig 6-4)

   a. Components
      Collar = 1, 2, 3, 4, 5 mm
      Abutment = 3.7 mm axial height
      Cement space = .75 mm
      Gold occlusal = 1.0 mm
      Ceramo-metal occlusal = 1.5–2.0 mm
      Ceramic core = .5 mm minimum

   b. CeraOne: gold occlusal
      1-mm CeraOne
      (abut. collar) = 1 mm
      abut. ht. above collar = 3.7 mm
      cement space = 0.75 mm
      gold occlusal = 1.0 mm
      _____
      total vertical height = 6.5 mm

   c. CeraOne: metal ceramic
      1-mm CeraOne
      (abut. collar) = 1 mm
      abutment ht.
      above collar = 3.7 mm
      cement space = 0.75 mm
      ceramo-mtl ocl. post. = 2.0 mm
      _____
      total vertical height = 7.5 mm

4. Minimum vertical space required is measured from the top of the implant to the occlusal contact of the opposing dentition.

Vertical Space Required	
Abutment	*Minimum Space*
EsthetiCone (1 mm)	6.7 mm
CeraOne (1 mm)	6.5 mm
CerAdapt	7.0 mm
Gold Cylinder to Fixture	2.8 mm

6

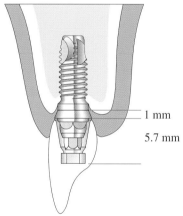

1 mm

5.7 mm

Fig 6-3

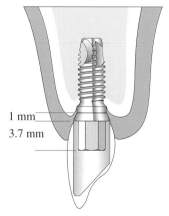

1 mm

3.7 mm

Fig 6-4

Space requirements (continued)

    d. Inclination of adjacent teeth (Fig 6–5)

       1. The position of adjacent teeth must be evaluated on a radiograph. The roots of these teeth can prevent implant placement if they converge. For a 4-mm implant, a minimum 6.5-mm mesiodistal space is needed.

       2. Sometimes orthodontics are necessary to reposition the tooth root to provide an adequate site for implant placement. If orthodontics are undertaken, the clinician should anticipate a possible buccolingual narrowing of the ridge as the teeth are moved.

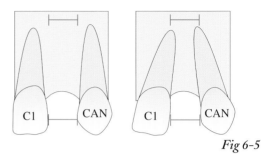

Fig 6-5

4. Risks of implant-supported single-tooth replacement

    a. Dark interdental areas (Fig 6–6)

    When a tooth is lost, there is often loss of the interdental papilla. Simply placing an implant and a crown does not replace the lost papilla. Only surgical manipulation of the hard and soft tissue-supporting structures can accomplish this goal. Many oral surgeons and periodontists consider the replacement of interdental papilla an unpredictable procedure. (The clinician should evaluate this area prior to surgery with a diagnostic wax-up or wax try-in.)

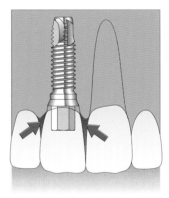

Fig 6-6

    b. Metal components show through (Fig 6–7)

    In a patient with a labially placed implant and thin translucent tissue, the metal components may show through.

    Prior to implant placement the clinician should note if the tissue is visible when the patient smiles. The thickness and translucency of the tissue should be evaluated.

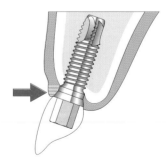

Fig 6-7

c. Adjacent single-tooth implants (Fig 6–8)

1. Multiple adjacent implants restored as single teeth should be avoided.

2. There is often difficulty in placing the restoration and simultaneously achieving proximal contacts.

3. If the implants are not close to being parallel to each other, insertion may not be possible.

4. With adjacent single tooth restorations the clinician is unable to fill-in or simulate the lost interdental papilla between the crowns. (Fig 6–9)

5. The dynamics of the multiple single-implant restoration are different than the multiple implant fixed partial denture. With single crowns, each restoration absorbs the occlusal load independently. A fixed partial denture (supported by several implants) distributes some of the load throughout the entire restoration and multiple implants.

5. Abutment selection

a. The crown-abutment interface in esthetic regions should be 2 to 3 mm below the free gingival margin. This is important for the maxillary anteriors and premolars when the patient has a high smile line.

b. Prior to abutment selection, the clinician can place a guide pin or direction indicator to evaluate the implant angulation. (Fig 6–10)

If the guide pin shows the long axis of the implant is to pass through the labial or facial surface, a cemented crown must be used. If it is on the lingual or palatal for an anterior tooth, a screw-retained or cemented restoration may be used.

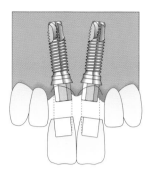

Fig 6-8

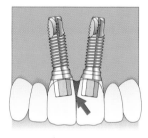

Fig 6-9

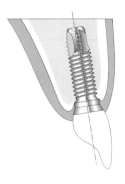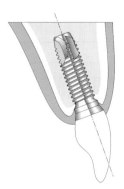

Fig 6-10

6

Single Tooth Replacement

1. Maxillary anterior
2. Maxillary premolar
3. Mandibular anterior
4. Mandibular premolar
5. Molar

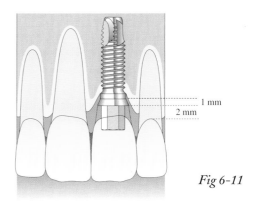

Fig 6-11

▼ Maxillary Anterior

1. Implant placement[3]
   a. The superior-inferior height of the implant should be 2 mm minimum above neighboring free gingival margin. The crown-abutment interface will be 1 mm below the free gingival margin with a 1 mm height abutment. (Fig 6–11)
   b. If the implant is not 2 mm above free gingival margin, problems result.
      1. Metal may show inadequate tissue depth to cover it.
      2. A short clinical crown may result, in comparison to the neighboring natural teeth. (Fig 6–12)
   c. For younger patients, the clinician should consider the potential for attachment loss and subsequent gingival recession. The implant should be placed higher (more superiorly) in the maxilla.

2. Labial inclination[3]
   a. Proper labial inclination is between the incisal edge and cingulum. (Fig 6–13)
   b. A compromised inclination of the implant with the long axis through the labial portion of tooth can often be avoided with surgical guide use. (Fig 6–14)
   c. If the implant emerges superior to the adjacent free gingival margins, a longer prosthetic tooth with poor esthetics results.

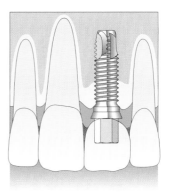

Fig 6-12

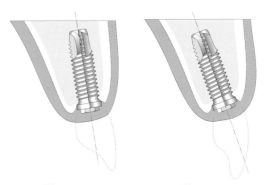

Fig 6-13   *Fig 6-14*

3. Labiolingual position

   a. Often with loss of tooth there is also loss of labial alveolar bone resulting in a concavity of the residual ridge. (Fig 6–15)

   b. When the implant is placed it is often positioned palatally. (Fig 6–16)

   c. The result is a cantilever labially creating simulated gingival margin. This often occurs with maxillary lateral incisors. The clinician should attempt to minimize the distance cantilevered facially. (Fig 6–17)

   d. With a concavity consider augmentation with:

      1. Soft tissue: to improve soft-tissue contours and esthetics

      2. Bone: to improve implant placement and resulting esthetics (Fig 6–18)

   e. The concavity may compromise incisogingival length of tooth, and esthetics.[3] If the augmentation is not done, then a long tooth results. (Fig 6–19)

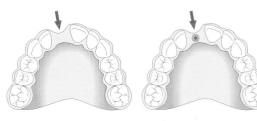

Fig 6-15   Fig 6-16

6

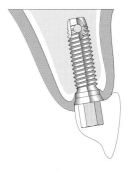
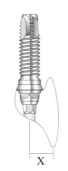

Fig 6-17

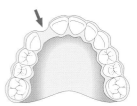
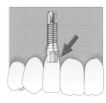

Fig 6-18   Fig 6-19

4. Site preparation

Augmentation of the ridge prior to implant placement can positively influence the restorative esthetics and biomechanics. (Figs 6–20 and 6–21)

5. Ridge width

Inadequate labiolingual ridge width often occurs with missing maxillary incisors (especially with congenitally missing maxillary lateral incisors). (Fig 6–22)

In some patients, there is not only a labial concavity but an inadequate labiolingual width of bone for implant placement. It is often necessary to augment the ridge width to permit implants. The alternative is no implant placement. (Fig 6–23)

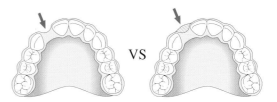

Fig 6-20

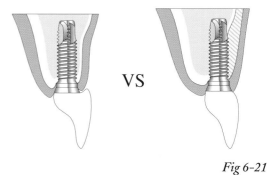

Fig 6-21

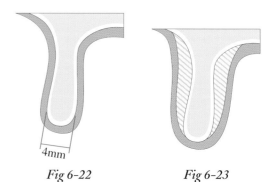

Fig 6-22   *Fig 6-23*

6. Occlusion

Prior to implant placement, the clinician must analyze the occlusal demands on the region.

a. Amount of vertical overlap: Some clinicians consider deep vertical overlap situations to contraindicate single-tooth implants.

b. Parafunctional habits: Increase the demands on the screw joint retaining the abutment. Some clinicians consider this a contraindication to single-tooth implants.

c. Contacts:

1. In casual intercuspation, the restoration may have slightly lighter contact than the rest of the dentition. In maximum intercuspation the single-tooth restoration should have simultaneous contact with the opposing natural dentition. Ideally, in excursive movements, the single-implant restoration should not be in contact.

2. The goal is to avoid placing the occlusal load solely on the single-tooth implant restoration.

3. The result should at least have simultaneous contact with the anterior implant tooth and neighboring natural teeth in excursions.

4. This may be especially difficult to create for the single missing maxillary cuspid. It is challenging to achieve contact simultaneously with implant and natural teeth and create a restoration that has an incisogingival length that harmonizes with the rest of the dentition.

d. A diagnostic wax-up with a denture tooth or inlay wax of the tooth is the best method to simulate the proposed restorative occlusal scheme. The protrusive and laterotrusive movements can be simulated while the shape and contour of the planned restoration is refined.

6

▼ Maxillary Premolar

1. There is often a buccal concavity of the ridge due to tooth loss. (Fig 6–24)

2. If implant is placed palatally (Fig 6–25), the restoration is cantilevered facially. A lever arm may thus be created, increasing the force on the components. (Fig 6–26)

3. There is often significant bone loss in the vertical direction. If the implant is placed in this situation a longer tooth (occluso-gingivally) may result (when viewed form the facial). This tooth does not harmonize with the height of the neighboring teeth. (Fig 6–27)

4. Site preparation often prevents this problem. The goal is augmentation with bone, or with bone and soft tissue simultaneously. (Fig 6–28)

   This allows optimal implant placement for the surgeon and better esthetics for the restorative dentist. (Fig 6–29)

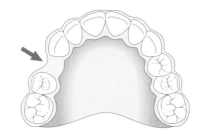

Fig 6-24

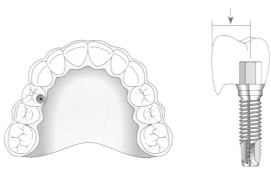

Fig 6-25   Fig 6-26

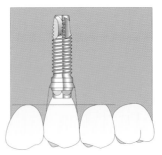

Fig 6-27

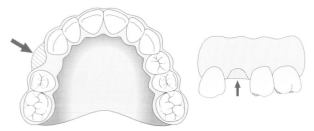

Fig 6-28   Fig 6-29

▼ Mandibular Anterior

1. Space limitation[1,2]
   a. To replace a missing single mandibular incisor is often challenging owing to the mesiodistal width of the space. (Fig 6–30)
   b. The width of the mandibular incisor is 4.5 mm to 5.5 mm mesiodistally. The edentulous space is often smaller as a result of overlap or drift of neighboring teeth. A mesiodistal space of 6.5 mm to 7 mm is needed to facilitate placement.[2]
   c. In some patients, single implants are not possible for single missing mandibular incisors due to insufficient mesiodistal space for components.
   d. There is also a problem with adequate labiolingual width of bone in this region. A minimum of 6 mm is needed but in cross-section the ridge is sometimes narrower.

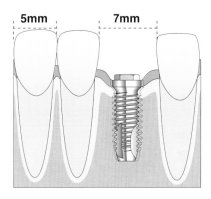

Fig 6-30

▼ Mandibular Premolar

1. The limiting factor for placement of an implant for mandibular premolar may be the position of the mental nerve, foramen, and loop. (Fig 6–31)

   There is often inadequate vertical height of bone superior to the nerve to allow for implant placement. Treatment options are:
   a. No implant
   b. Surgical repositioning of the neurovascular bundle
      1. Surgical risks do exist with this procedure.
      2. The surgeon and the patient should carefully consider the risks and benefits of this procedure.

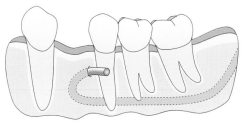

Fig 6-31

▼ Molar

1. Considerations
   a. Some clinicians consider single-tooth replacement to be contraindicated for molars because the size of the occlusal surface and the number of contacts during function place huge loads on the components. The screw joint is particularly at risk. Even the bone-implant interface is challenged in some patients.

   b. Prior to implant placement, the clinician should measure the mesiodistal space to be restored. (Fig 6–32)

   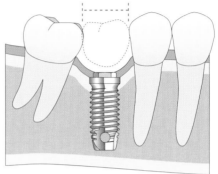

   Fig 6-32

   1. If there has been mesial drift of the second molar, the occlusal demand of the implant restoration may lessen due to the decreased mesiodistal space to be restored. The restoration may be only the size of a premolar, but a more predictable restoration is the result.

   2. The clinician should not necessarily perform orthodontics and move the second molar distally. This will create a molar-sized space, but may result in a less predictable restoration.

   c. The buccolingual width of the bone needed is 6 mm. This allows placement of a 4-mm-wide implant with 1 mm of bone on each side. Use of the 3.75-mm fixture has been identified in some fixture fractures for single molars[4] and should be avoided.

   d. The clinician should consider the individual restorative situation: for example, a patient with a single missing first molar; a second premolar with a large existing restoration; and a second molar with a large restoration or carious lesion. A conventional three-unit partial denture retained by natural teeth is optimal, because the teeth on either side require restoration.

2. Limitations

    a. For a single missing maxillary molar, the limiting factor is the vertical bone height below the maxillary sinus.

    b. For a single missing mandibular molar, the limiting factor is the bone height above the inferior alveolar nerve.

3. Position

    a. Center the implant mesiodistally, to direct the force on the implant along the long axis. (Fig 6–33)

    b. If the implant is positioned to the mesial or distal, a cantilever is created (Fig 6–34), which tends to open the screw joint and loosen or fracture the screw.[5,6] (Fig 6–35)

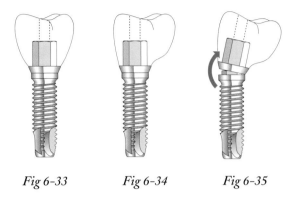

Fig 6-33   Fig 6-34   Fig 6-35

4. Number of implants

    a. Some clinicians suggest placing two implants to replace the missing roots of the molar. Owing to anatomical limitations, this cannot be accomplished in all situations. (Fig 6–36)

       1. The mesiodistal space between the natural teeth may not allow placement of two implants.

       2. It is technically difficult to fit components in some clinical situations. Often the gold cylinders cannot be seated due to implant angulation and proximity to each other.

         If only one implant is possible a wider implant is necessary (4 mm or 5 mm).

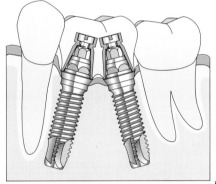

Fig 6-36

    b. When the single missing tooth is the most distal molar, the clinician should use two implants rather than one. Two implants are generally considered for missing molars because the occlusal demands are high. Often, if it is the most distal tooth, there is available bone for multiple implant placement. (Fig 6–37)

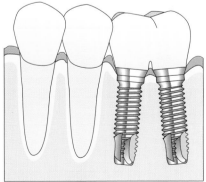

Fig 6-37

6

5. Fabrication of the restoration

  a. Narrowing the occlusal surface buccolingually will reduce the occlusal load on the restoration.[5] (Fig 6–38)

  b. Flattening the cusps of the restoration has been suggested to reduce the occlusal load in the horizontal direction.[5] (Fig 6–39)

  c. Ideally, in laterotrusion and protrusion, the molar single-tooth replacement should be out of occlusion to guard against overloading. This is most important for patients with parafunctional habits.

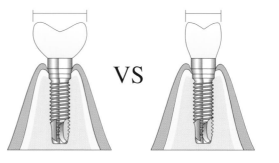

Fig 6-38

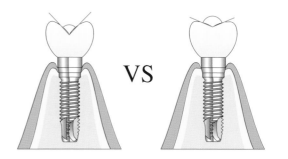

Fig 6-39

Patient Presentations

1. Patient 1
   a. Tooth 10 was lost due to a perforation of the root with a custom cast post and core. A vertical bony defect resulted and the tooth was removed. (Fig 6–40)
   b. An osseointegrated implant was placed in position 10. Second stage surgery with a definitive abutment placement has been accomplished. (Fig 6–41)
   c. Tooth 10 has an osseointegrated implant restored with a CeraOne abutment and a metal ceramic cemented restoration. Teeth 11 through 15 have been restored with metal ceramic restorations on natural teeth. (Fig 6–42)

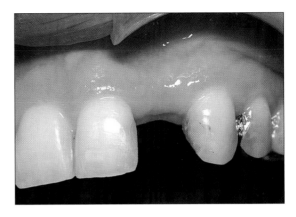

Fig 6-40

6

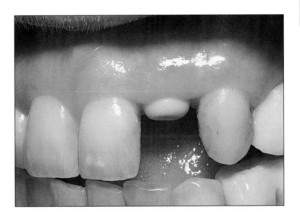

Fig 6-41

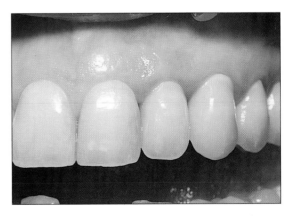

Fig 6-42

Surgery by Dr Neil Hagen
Laboratory procedures by Toshihiro Takasaki

2. Patient 2

   a. The patient has lost tooth 9 due to a traumatic blow. (Fig 6–43)

   b. Tooth 9 is missing and there is loss of labial and palatal bone and supporting structures. This defect requires augmentation in addition to implant placement. (Fig 6–44)

   c. A chin graft was placed into the defect and allowed to heal. The implant was placed at a second surgery and allowed to osseointegrate for six months. The final restoration included a CeraOne abutment placed and a cemented metal ceramic restoration. (Fig 6–45)

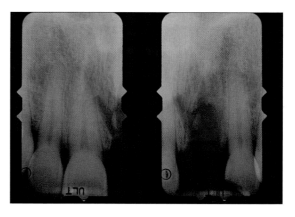

Fig 6-43

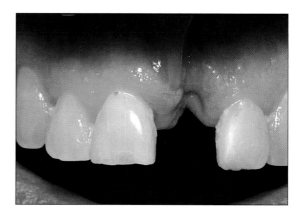

Fig 6-44

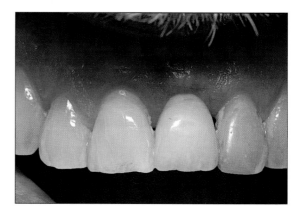

Fig 6-45

Surgery by Dr Michael Stohle

Laboratory procedures by Toshihiro Takasaki

3. Patient 3
   a. Tooth 5 is missing on this patient and a single osseointegrated implant was placed with a CeraOne abutment. Notice that the occlusal aspect of the implant is below the cemento-enamel junction of the anticipated free gingival margin by several millimeters. This allows a normal occlusogingival height of the restoration. (Fig 6–46)
   b. Definitive restoration is a metal ceramic restoration cemented on a CeraOne abutment. (Fig 6–47)

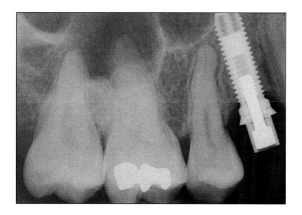

Fig 6-46

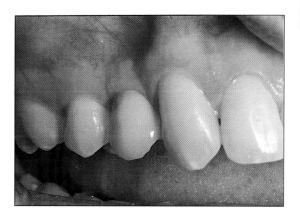

Fig 6-47

6

Surgery by Dr Michael Stohle
Laboratory procedures by Toshihiro Takasaki

4. Patient 4

   a. A single missing molar is a challenging restoration for an implant because the mesiodistal space is 10 to 12 mm. Tooth 19 is missing and the mesiodistal space is inadequate for two implants. One osseointegrated implant was placed with a CeraOne abutment. (Fig 6–48)

   b. Definitive metal ceramic restoration cemented in place. (Fig 6–49)

   c. Note that the buccolingual width of the restoration has been narrowed slightly in order to reduce the amount of stress on the restoration. Also not that the centric contact has been centralized or placed toward the center of the tooth, over the implant. This allows for less bending movement and tends to place the force in the vertical axis of the implant. (Fig 6–50)

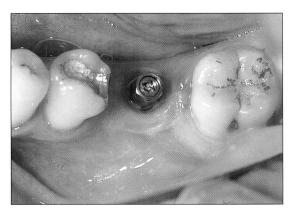

Fig 6-48

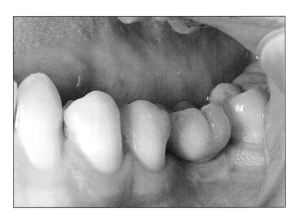

Fig 6-49

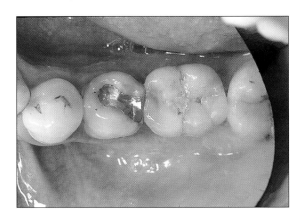

Fig 6-50

Surgery by Dr Todd Jensen
Laboratory procedures by Toshihiro Takasaki

5. Patient 5

   a. The patient has lost tooth 18. Tooth 15 has drifted into edentulous space. The treatment plan is for two implants because there is adequate mesiodistal space. This is also the last molar in the area so two implants are the treatment of choice. (Fig 6–51)

   b. The definitive restoration is a two-unit fixed partial denture. This restoration utilized MirusCone abutments and gold cylinders. The mesial portion is fabricated as a metal ceramic restoration and the distal portion is a cast metal gold cylinder. (Fig 6–52)

   c. Occlusal view of the restoration on tooth in place 18 supported by two implants. (Fig 6–53)

   d. Buccal view of the final restoration in place with a metal ceramic crown on tooth 15 and the implant-supported, two-unit fixed partial denture on tooth 18. (Fig 6–54)

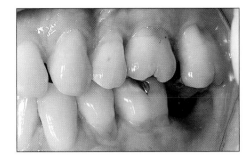

Fig 6-51

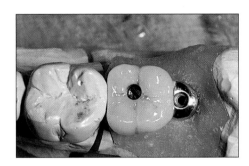

Fig 6-52

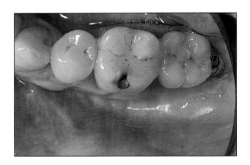

Fig 6-53

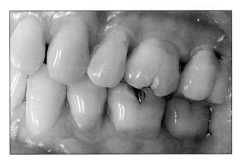

Fig 6-54

6

Surgery by Dr Richard Martino
Laboratory procedures by Toshihiro Takasaki

References

1. Ohrnell L, Palmquist J, Brånemark PI. Single tooth replacement. In: Worthington P, Brånemark PI, eds. Advanced Osseointegration Surgery: Applications in the Maxillofacial Region. Chicago: Quintessence; 1992:211–232.

2. Lekholm U, Jemt T. Principles for single tooth replacement. In: Albrektsson T, Zarb GA, eds. The Brånemark Osseointegrated Implant. Chicago: Quintessence; 1989:117–126.

3. Parel S, Sullivan D. Esthetics and Osseointegration. Dallas: Taylor; 1989:11–12, 20–21.

4. Rangert B, Krogh P, Langer B. Bending overload and implant fracture: A retrospective clinical analysis. Int J Oral Maxillofac Implants 1995;10:326–334.

5. Jorneus L. Avoiding overload in single tooth restorations. Nobelpharma News 1992;4:3.

6. Rangert B. Biomechanical considerations for partial prosthesis. Nobelpharma News 1992;6:2:4.

7

Partially Edentulous Considerations

The restoration of partially edentulous patients in general requires attention to concepts that are not considered with the restoration of natural teeth. The restoration of the partially edentulous patient with implants is different in some respects from restoration with conventional dentistry.

General Concepts

1. Uniting multiple implants
   a. Multiple implants should be splinted. The result is a mechanical advantage at the screw level. (Fig 7–1)

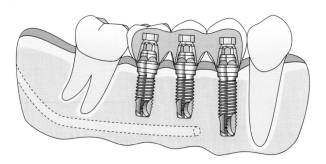

Fig 7-1

2. Mesiodistal placement

   a. The ideal implant placement is in the center of the occlusal surface mesiodistally for more optimal esthetics and loading of components.[1] (Fig 7–2)

   b. The surgeon should avoid placement in the interproximal region. Interproximal placement makes it very difficult for both the restorative dentist and the technician to create normal emergence profiles and esthetics.

3. Buccolingual placement[1]

   a. Ideal placement is in the center of the occlusal surface buccolingually. This places the force primarily in the long axis of the implant. It also reduces the cantilever effect buccally or lingually and thus reduces the bending moment. Implants placed to the lingual create a lever arm or cantilever to the buccal, which amplifies the load on the components. (Fig 7–3)

4. Tripod

   a. Ideally, multiple implants are slightly staggered or tripoded to provide better support. Thus three implants, because they can be tripoded, have a mechanical advantage over two implants. Three implants tripoded have an advantage over three implants in a straight line.[2] (Fig 7–4)

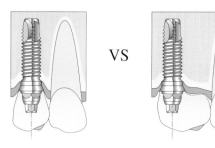

Fig 7-2

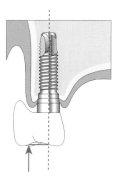

Fig 7-3

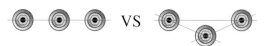

Fig 7-4

b. If a three-unit fixed prosthesis is restored with the implants at each end, a stress value of 100% can be established. If a two-implant prosthesis has a cantilever, the stress is doubled. For the three-unit prosthesis with a third implant added, the stress is reduced by one third. If the three implants are tripoded, the total stress is one third of the original two-implant, three-unit prosthesis. The importance of implant placement and number of implants in preventing overload is critical.(Fig 7–5; from Rangert.[3] Used with permission)

5. Axial load[4]

a. The ideal is to load the implant along its long axis. (Fig 7–6) Implants placed at an angle and restored have an increase in shear force on the components. The clinician should be conservative in the design of the restoration on the angulated implant.

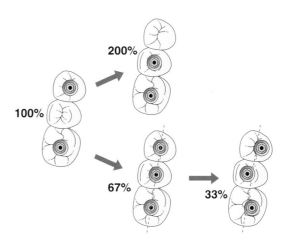

100%

200%

67%

33%

Fig 7-5

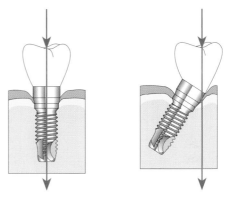

Fig 7-6

7

6. Vertical space (Fig 7–7)

   a. The minimum vertical space needed, from the superior aspect of the implant to the opposing occlusion, depends on the abutment selected.

   b. The clinician should measure this space on the mounted diagnostic casts. The soft tissue has some thickness so the space is larger than measured. The thickness in the mandibular arch can be estimated at about 1 mm and in the maxillary arch at about 2 mm.

   c. Prior to implant placement, the clinician should analyze the vertical space and the plane of occlusion. If inadequate space is available, there are several options:

      1. Enameloplasty or occlusal adjustment of opposing dentition

      2. Restore the opposing dentition

      3. Orthodontics

      4. Segmental osteotomy plus orthodontics (Fig 7–8)

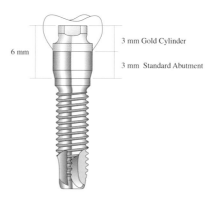

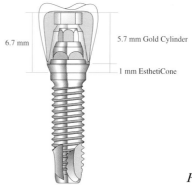

Fig 7-7

Vertical Space Required	
Abutment	*Minimum Space*
Standard (3 mm)	6.0 mm
EsthetiCone (1 mm)	6.7 mm
Mirus Cone (1 mm)	4.5 mm
Angulated 30° (4 mm)	8.5 mm
Angulated 17° (2 mm)	7.4 mm
Gold Cylinder to Fixture	2.8 mm

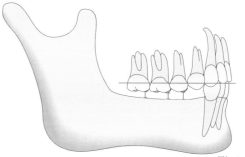

Fig 7-8

7. Distance between implants

a. The distance between implants, center to center, must be 7 mm (with 3.75- or 4-mm implants). This leaves 3 mm of vital bone between implant surfaces or 1.5 mm of bone surrounding each implant. (Fig 7–9)

b. If a wider implant is utilized, this distance must be increased. When a 5-mm implant is used, the distance should be 8 mm center to center.

8. Distance from implant to natural tooth

a. The distance from implant to natural tooth varies depending on the inclination of the adjacent tooth. The clinician should evaluate the patient's radiographs carefully. (Fig 7–10)

b. In some situations the natural tooth is in the same long axis as the planned implant axis. The goals are to retain vital bone around the tooth and implant, and to avoid violating the periodontal ligament and natural tooth. With a 3.75- or 4-mm implant: if the distance from the implant center to the proximal aspect of the tooth (x) is 4 mm, there is at least 2 mm of vital bone and periodontal ligament between tooth and implant. (Fig 7–11) But, often the tooth is inclined toward the edentulous space. The planned implant then must be inclined or moved further away from the natural tooth to provide adequate vital bone around the implant and natural tooth.

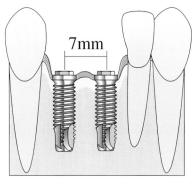

Fig 7-9

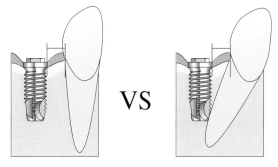

Fig 7-10

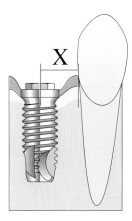

Fig 7-11

9. Determining number of implants to be utilized[5]

a. Measure mesiodistal width of the edentulous space between the proximal tooth surfaces. Some clinicians use the following formula for 3.75- or 4-mm implants:

$$\frac{(x-1 \text{ mm})}{7} = \text{\# of implants}$$

where x = the mesiodistal width of the space. (Fig 7–12)

b. If x ≥ 22 mm, 3 implants are possible.
   If x ≥ 15 mm, 2 implants are possible.
   If x < 15 mm, 1 implant is possible. (Fig 7–13)

10. Ridge width

a. The clinician should confirm a 6-mm width ridge for the 3.75- or 4-mm implants. This allows 1 mm of vital bone on the facial and lingual surface of the implant.

11. Abutment selection

a. The location of the abutment-gold cylinder interface for sublingual components has been suggested to be 2 to 3 mm from the free gingival margin on the facial side in an esthetically critical area. (Fig 7–14)

b. This provides for 2 to 3 mm of the crown to be subgingival and allows the clinician to place the porcelain-metal junction subgingivally.

c. If this interface is placed too far subgingivally, placement of the restoration is more difficult. Maintaining the soft-tissue contour during the restorative procedures is challenging with a deep collar of tissue.

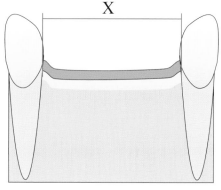

Fig 7-12

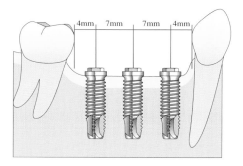

Fig 7-13

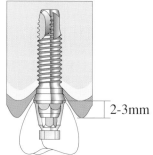

Fig 7-14

Example

Tissue Depth (mm)	Abutment Height (mm)
3	1
4	1
5	2
6	3

   d. The soft-tissue depth differs at various positions around the implant. This is especially true in the maxilla. (Fig 7–15)

   e. Many components are useful in improving esthetics because the abutment-gold cylinder interface is subgingival. In some situations, the clinician may want to have the abutment at the soft-tissue margin. This often occurs in the mandibular posterior region where esthetics are not an issue. The advantage of sublingual interfaces in the mandibular posterior is a more natural emergence profile that facilitates daily maintenance and discourages debris accumulation.

12. Timing of definitive abutment placement

   a. The restorative goal is placement when the surrounding tissue has matured. The restorative dentist should wait for soft tissue healing. This time period ranges from 30 to 90 days after the second surgery. The healing abutment is left in place for at least one month to allow soft tissue healing.

   b. Then, the definitive abutment is placed. After this healing period, final impressions can be made. If they are made too early, gingival contours are less predictable. For highly esthetic regions, the clinician must wait longer to assure soft tissue maturity.

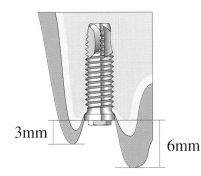

3mm   6mm

Fig 7-15

7

13. Provisionalization[6] (Fig 7–16)

   a. Provisionalization plays an important role prior to definitive restoration fabrication. The purpose of the provisional restoration is:

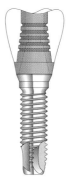

Fig 7-16

     1. To develop embrasure form, contour, and esthetics of the definitive restoration.

     2. To create the desired emergence contour of the restoration through the soft tissue by influencing the soft tissue contour during healing.

     3. To determine occlusal scheme.

     4. To determine the inter-arch distance (VDO—vertical dimension of occlusion).

     5. To provide a fixed restoration during soft tissue healing.

     6. To prevent movement of the opposing or neighboring teeth during fabrication of the restoration. This is especially important after orthodontic treatment.

     7. To educate the patient about the limitations of their specific clinical situation.

     8. To provide for incremental loading. Some clinicians suggest this is most useful for the maxillary posterior partially edentulous patient. (See Chapter 9.)

     9. To increase treatment time. This may help the patient distribute the cost over a longer period of time.

14. Restoration fabrication

a. The clinician should fabricate the implant restoration with an occlusal table narrower (buccolingually) than the natural teeth being replaced, to reduce force to the components. (Fig 7–17)

15. Tooth-implant connection[7-17]

a. Situation (Fig 7–18)

1. There is a difference in mobility of implant and natural tooth owing to the lack of a periodontal ligament surrounding the implant.[7] If the implant is connected to a natural tooth, the prosthesis is a long cantilever off the implant. With a rigid connection, the implant carries the majority of the occlusal load when the tooth moves.

2. The interfaces between the metal components also have some mobility under function.[8] (Fig 7–19)

3. There is some flexibility of the screws used to retain the components.[8]

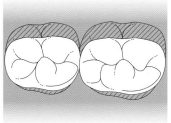

Fig 7-17

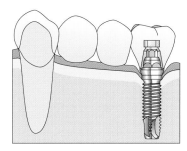

Fig 7-18

7

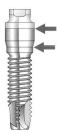

Fig 7-19

Tooth–implant connections (continued)

b. Options

  1. Separate

    a. Ideally, the clinician should restore the implants independent of the natural tooth—thus more implants should be placed. The goal is one implant per missing tooth for posterior fixed partial dentures. This cannot be achieved for every patient. (Fig 7–20)

  2. Non-rigid connector (Fig 7–21)

    a. Advantage

      • The clinician can retrieve the implant portion of the restoration without disturbing the natural tooth.

    b. Disadvantages (Fig 7–22)

      • Uneven marginal ridges between the implant crown and the natural tooth crown appear over time.

      • Loosening of the gold screw is more frequent.

      • Intrusion of natural tooth has been reported.

      • The clinician must restore the natural tooth with resulting periodontal, endodontic, and caries risks.

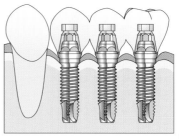

Fig 7-20

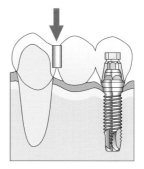

Fig 7-21

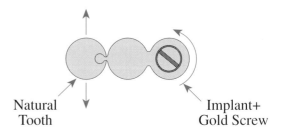

Natural Tooth   Implant+ Gold Screw

Fig 7-22

3. Telescopic coping (Fig 7–23)

  a. Disadvantages

    • Multiple layers exist above the preparation of the natural tooth including:

        Luting agent

        Telescopic coping

        Metal framework of the fixed partial denture (FPD)

        Porcelain (if porcelain occlusal)

    • Often the natural tooth is reduced inadequately, resulting in thinner components and weakening of the prosthesis. The metal of the FPD fractures at the natural tooth.

    • When the natural tooth is reduced excessively, endodontic treatment is necessary.

    • A decision on luting agent between the coping and partial denture must be made. Restorative options include:

        Nothing

        Silicone

        Temporary cement

        Permanent luting agent (If permanent luting agent is used, retrievability is reduced)

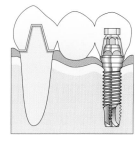

Fig 7-23

4. T-block, screw, or U-pin (Fig 7–24)

  a. Advantages

    • The retrievability is preserved.

  b. Disadvantages

    • The implant crown is still united to the natural tooth.

    • A cantilever is still created off of the implant when the natural tooth moves.

    • This option is more technically challenging.

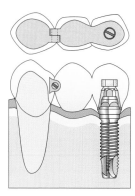

Fig 7-24

7

111

Tooth–implant connections/Options (continued)

    5. Double abutment of natural teeth (Fig 7–25)

       a. Advantage

- There is more optimal force distribution when two natural teeth are splinted together and then united with an implant.

       b. Disadvantages

- A cantilever off the implant is still created when the natural teeth move.
- When multiple teeth and multiple implants are splinted together there is a possibility of the tooth migrating out from under the partial denturework. A space is then created between the restoration margin and the tooth.

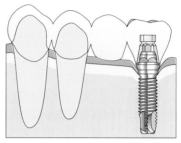

Fig 7-25

16. Number of implants

    a. Posterior fixed partial dentures with two implants have been shown to be inferior to those supported by three or more implants.

      1. With three implants the clinician can tripod the placement resulting in a more stable prosthesis.[3]

      2. More mechanical problems occur with two-implant prostheses than with three-implant prostheses.[19,20]

      3. Two-implant prostheses are at higher risk for implant fracture than are three-implant prostheses.[21]

References

1. Rangert B, Jemt T, Jorneus L. Forces and moments on Brånemark implants. Int J Oral Maxillofac Implants 1989;4:241–247.

2. Rangert B. Biomechanical considerations for partial prosthesis. Nobelpharma News 1992;6(2):4–5.

3. Rangert B, Sullivan R. Learning from history: The transition from full arch to posterior partial restorations. Nobelpharma News 1995;9(2):6–7.

4. Kinni M, Hokama S, Caputo A. Force transfer by osseointegration implant devices. Int J Oral Maxillofac Implants 1987;2:1:11–14.

5. Jemt T. Restoration of osseointegrated implants. Lecture for Chicago Dental Society; Midwinter Meeting, 1992; Chicago, IL.

6. Emerson J. The provisional implant restoration. Esthetic Dent Update 1993;4:89–92.

7. Sekine H, Komiyama Y, Hotta H, Yoshida K. Mobility characters and tactile sensitivity of osseointegrated fixture-supporting system in tissue integration; oral and maxillofacial reconstruction. Amsterdam Excerpta Medica 1986;326–332.

8. Rangert B, Gunne J, Sullivan D. Mechanical aspects of a Brånemark implant connected to a natural tooth: An in-vitro study. Int J Oral Maxillofac Implants 1991;6:177–186.

9. Astrand P, Borg K, Gunne J, Olsson M. Combination of natural teeth and osseointegrated implants as prosthesis abutments: A 2-year study. Int J Oral Maxillofac Implants 1991;6:305–312.

10. Ericsson I, Lekholm U, Brånemark PI, Lindhe J, Nyman S. A clinical evaluation of fixed-partial denture restorations supported by the combination of teeth and osseointegrated implants. Int J Oral Maxillofac Implants 1986;13:307–312.

11. Ericsson I, Glantz P, Brånemark PI. Use of implants in restorative therapy in patients with reduced periodontal tissue support. Quintessence Int 1988;19:801–807.

12. Reider C, Parel S. A survey of natural tooth abutment intrusion with implant-connected fixed partial dentures. Int J Periodont Res Dent 1993;13:335–347.

13. Langer B, Sullivan D. Osseointegration: Its impact on the interrelationship of periodontics and restorative dentistry: Part II. Int J Periodont Res Dent 1989;9:165–183.

14. Sheets C, Earthman JC. Natural tooth intrusion and reversal in implant assisted prosthesis. J Prosthet Dent 1993;70:513–520.

15. Sullivan D. Prosthetic considerations for the utilization of osseointegrated fixtures in the partially edentulous arch. Int J Oral Maxillofac Implants 1986;1:39–45.

16. Cho G, Chee W. Apparent intrusion of natural teeth under an implant—supported prosthesis: A clinical report. J Prosthet Dent 1992;68:3–5.

17. Gunne J. A longitudinal study of partial dentures supported by both implants & natural teeth. Clin Oral Implant Res 1992;3:49–56.

18. Ericsson I, Brånemark PI, Glatz P. Partial edentulism. In: Worthington P, Brånemark PI, eds. Advanced Osseointegration Surgery. Chicago: Quintessence; 1992:194–209.

19. Lekholm U, van Steenberghe D, Herrmann I. Osseointegrated implants in the treatment of partially edentulous jaws: A prospective 5-year multi-center study. Int J Oral Maxillofac Implants 1994;9:627–635.

20. Jemt T, Lekholm U. Oral implants in posterior partially edentulous jaws: A 5-year follow-up study. Int J Oral Maxillofac Implants 1993;8:635–640.

21. Rangert B, Krogh P, Langer B. Bending overload and implant fracture: A retrospective clinical analysis. Int J Oral Maxillofac Implants 1995;10:326–334.

7

Maxillary Anterior— Partially Edentulous

Goal

1. Fixed prosthesis
2. Restoration independent of natural teeth

Presurgical Needs

1. Mounted diagnostic casts
2. Diagnostic wax-up, denture teeth, or full-contour wax-up
3. Surgical guide—critical
   a. The surgical guide can be coated with a radiopaque material (barium sulfate) and worn during the computerized axial tomograms.
   b. The resulting image is useful in evaluating the relationship between the available bone and the proposed position of the prosthetic tooth.
4. Examination of high smile line—critical
5. Radiographs
   a. Full-mouth periapicals to analyze prognosis of existing natural teeth
   b. Panoramic radiograph
   c. Tomogram to analyze bone width and height
   d. Computerized axial tomogram to analyze bone width and height
   e. Occlusal film to determine location and size of incisive canal
6. Wax try-in of denture teeth on record base with no labial flange to show where the prosthetic tooth placement is in relation to the residual ridge.

Considerations

1. Crossing midline[1]
   a. If the partially edentulous space crosses the midline, the clinician should consider each segment to the right or left of the incisive canal separately. The position of the incisive canal limits implant placement. (Fig 8–1)

   b. On an occlusal film, the clinician should measure the distance from the proximal surface of the tooth to the lateral extent of the incisive canal. Using the formula (see page 106)

   $$\frac{x-1 \text{ mm}}{7} = \# \text{ of implants}$$

   where x = distance from the proximal tooth surface to the lateral extent of the incisive canal:

   1. If $x \geq 22$ mm, 3 implants are possible. (Fig 8–2)
   2. If $x \geq 15$ mm, 2 implants are possible. (Fig 8–3)
   3. If $x < 15$ mm, 1 implant is possible.

   c. This distance may also be estimated on a diagnostic cast.

2. Number of implants
   a. Often owing to the size and position of incisive papilla, only two implants are possible in the lateral incisor area when the four incisors are missing. Because of the reduced forces in the anterior region, this is an adequate number of implants. (Fig 8–4)

   b. When an edentulous space crosses midline, the clinician should consider it as two segments.

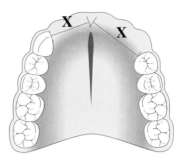

Fig 8-1

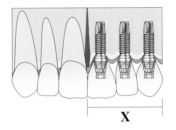

Fig 8-2

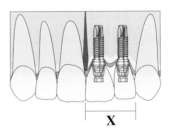

Fig 8-3

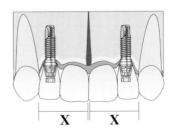

Fig 8-4

3. Vertical space limitation (Fig 8–5)

a. The vertical measurement from the maxillary residual ridge to the incisal edge of the mandibular anteriors should be noted. The standard components need 6 mm of vertical space (3 mm abutment plus 3 mm gold cylinder). The Estheti-Cone needs 6.7 mm of vertical space (1 mm abutment plus 5.7 mm gold cylinder). Note that soft-tissue thickness varies in this region, but it is often a minimum of 2-mm thick. The Mirus Cone allows a restoration in 4.5 mm of vertical space.

4. Labiolingual placement

a. The ideal screw-access hole is positioned between incisal edge and cingulum. (Fig 8–6)

b. Often the labial bone has been lost or has resorbed after extraction. The implant is then placed palatally. This occurs in the lateral incisor region due to a labial concavity. The restorative result is a ridge lap for simulation of a free gingival margin. (Fig 8–7)

c. The clinician should consider minimizing the anterior-labial cantilever. A lever arm has been created, increasing the force on the restoration.

d. Site preparation by augmenting with bone enhances implant placement for improved esthetics and biomechanical loading.

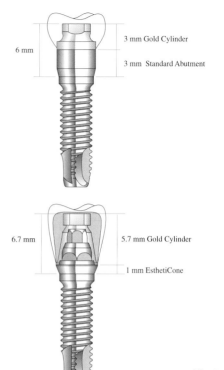

6 mm

3 mm Gold Cylinder

3 mm Standard Abutment

6.7 mm

5.7 mm Gold Cylinder

1 mm EsthetiCone

Fig 8-5

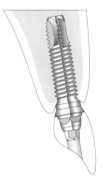

Fig 8-6

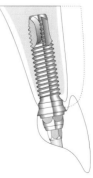

Fig 8-7

Vertical Space Required	
Abutment	*Minimum Space*
Standard (3 mm)	6.0 mm
EsthetiCone (1 mm)	6.7 mm
Mirus Cone (1 mm)	4.5 mm
Angulated 30° (4 mm)	8.5 mm
Angulated 17° (2 mm)	7.4 mm
Gold Cylinder to Fixture	2.8 mm

8

5. Residual ridge contour (Fig 8–8)

a. A labial concavity often results when a tooth and the labial bone are lost. Implants are placed more palatally, and the emergence of the restoration is difficult or a ridge lap results.

b. Tooth loss often results in vertical bone loss, which compromises the restoration. The result is a long tooth (Fig 8–9), which can be a significant esthetic problem with a high smile line.

c. In cross section (Fig 8–10), the lateral incisor region often has a labial concavity, which requires palatal implant position.

1. Ideally, surgical augmentation should be performed in addition to implant placement. (Fig 8–11)

2. In cross section, the labiolingual width is also often inadequate. (Fig 8–12)

3. The 4-mm-wide implant requires a 6-mm width of bone.

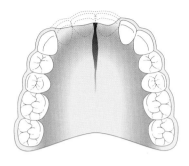

Fig 8-8

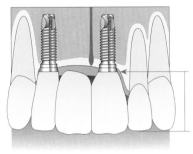

Fig 8-9

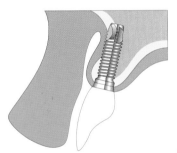

Fig 8-10

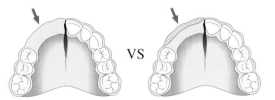

VS

Fig 8-11

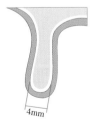

4mm

Fig 8-12

6. Implant placement

    a. Goal: Implant placement in the mesiodistal center of the proposed restorative tooth. (Fig 8–13)

    b. If the implant is placed interproximally, esthetics and emergence profile are compromised. (Fig 8–14) This is especially true with the maxillary anterior region and in a patient with a high smile line.

7. Presurgical esthetic evaluation (Fig 8–15)

    a. The planned position of the prosthetic tooth should be compared to the position and contour of the residual ridge. This can be evaluated with a wax try-in using denture teeth on a record base. The record base (baseplate) should be fabricated with no flange above the maxillary anterior teeth. The clinician can then analyze the proposed implant site.

    b. The patient profile should also be evaluated.

8. After second surgery

    a. The clinician should wait for soft-tissue healing, especially with a high smile, as tissue contour changes with time.

    b. The clinician should delay definitive abutment placement in this esthetically sensitive area. The healing abutment should remain in place for a minimum of four weeks of tissue healing.

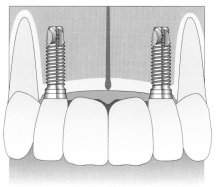

Fig 8-13

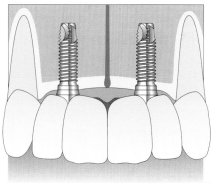

Fig 8-14

8

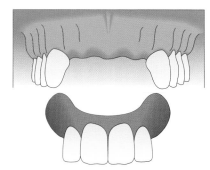

Fig 8-15

Patient Examples[7–10]

The following patient examples are intended to assist the restorative dentist in planning optimal implant placement. For some of the clinical situations several treatment options exist and the anticipated advantages and disadvantages are suggested. These are intended as guidelines only and the clinician must remember that each patient is unique with specific restorative requirements.

▼ Missing: Maxillary Left-Central and Lateral Incisors (Fig 8–16)

1. Considerations
   a. Position of incisive canal
   b. Mesiodistal width of space
   c. Buccolingual width of bone
   d. High smile line
   e. Labial contour of remaining ridge
      (Note: think three-dimensionally.)
   f. Vertical height of space
2. Plan
   a. Two-unit fixed partial denture with two implants: one for each tooth if there is adequate bone (if mesiodistal width > 15 mm).

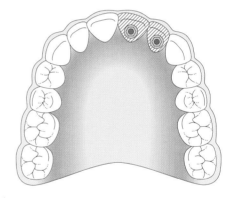

Fig 8-16

▼ Missing: Maxillary Left-Lateral Incisor and Canine (Fig 8–17)

1. Considerations
   a. Mesiodistal width of space
   b. Buccolingual width of bone
   c. High smile line
   d. Labial contour of residual ridge
   e. Vertical space available
   f. Occlusal scheme
2. Plan
   a. Two-unit fixed partial denture with two implants (if mesiodistal width > 15 mm).
   b. Augmentation may be necessary to create esthetic contours.
   c. The goal for the occlusal scheme should be simultaneous contact between teeth and implants.

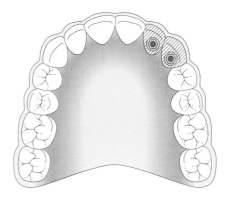

Fig 8-17

▼ Missing: Maxillary Central Incisors (Fig 8–18)

1. Considerations
   a. Position and size of incisive canal
   b. Mesiodistal width of space
   c. Buccolingual width of bone
   d. High smile line
   e. Labial contour of ridge
   f. Vertical space available
2. Plan
   (Note: use of two implants can be difficult owing to the size and position of the incisive canal.)
   a. Two implants and a two-unit fixed partial denture.

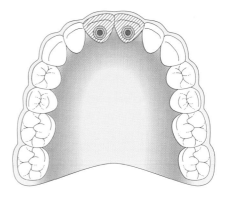

Fig 8-18

8

▼ Missing: Maxillary Left-Central and Lateral Incisor and Canine

(Fig 8–19)

1. Considerations
   a. Mesiodistal width of space
   b. Buccolingual width of bone
   c. High smile line
   d. Labial contour of ridge
   e. Vertical space available
2. Plan
   a. Two implants and a three-unit fixed partial denture
3. Alternative Plan
   a. One implant per tooth if there is adequate mesiodistal width (> 22 mm) and buccolingual bone

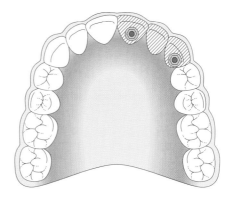

Fig 8-19

▼ Missing: Maxillary Central Incisors and Left Lateral Incisor

(Fig 8–20)

1. Considerations
   a. Mesiodistal width of space
   b. Buccolingual width of bone
   c. High smile line
   d. Position of incisive canal
      1. Treat right and left sides separately; measure space from lateral aspect of incisive canal to tooth on each side.
   e. Labial contour of ridge
   f. Vertical space available
2. Plan
   a. Three-unit fixed partial denture.
   b. Often only two implants are possible due to incisive canal position.
   c. If there is large space and bone allowance, three implants are possible.

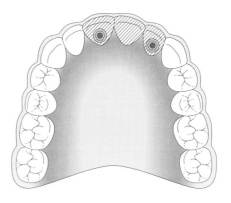

Fig 8-20

▼ Missing: Maxillary Central and Lateral Incisors (Fig 8–21)

1. Considerations
   a. Buccolingual width of ridge
   b. High smile line
   c. Labial ridge contour
   d. Position and size of incisive canal
      1. Treat right and left segments separately. Measure from lateral aspect of incisive canal to neighboring natural tooth.
   e. Vertical space available

2. Plan
   a. Two implants (lateral incisors) and four-unit partial denture.
   b. Often only two implants are possible due to the position of the incisive canal.
   c. The clinician may use additional implants in available bone.

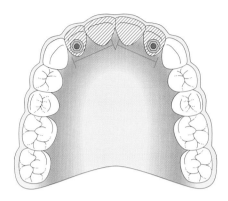

Fig 8-21

3. Alternative plan (Fig 8–22)
   a. Two implants (central incisors) and a four-unit partial denture.
      Note: one lateral incisor is cantilevered distally. This can be planned because there is less demand on this restoration than in the molar region for many patients.
   b. The clinician should analyze the occlusal scheme, parafunctional habits, opposing occlusion, and presence of posterior support.
   c. Avoid placement of implants interproximally.

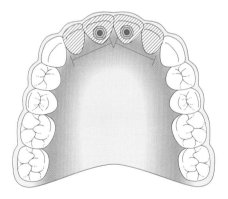

Fig 8-22

8

▼

▼ **Missing: Maxillary Central Incisors, Lateral Incisors, and Canines** (Fig 8–23)

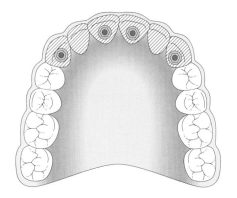

Fig 8-23

1. Considerations
   a. Ridge width
   b. High smile line
   c. Labial ridge contour
   d. Wax try-in prior to surgery
   e. Occlusal scheme
   f. Vertical space available
2. Plan
   a. Six-unit fixed partial denture.
   b. Four implants are often possible. Measurement of space should be done in two segments.
   c. Ridge augmentation is often required.

Patient Presentations

1. Patient 1
   a. As a result of a traumatic accident this patient has lost four teeth, 7 to 10. Two osseointegrated implants have been placed. Note that these implants are slightly angled toward the midline posing a difficult restorative situation. They were placed in the anticipated embrasures, which would normally be the narrowest portion of the restoration. (Fig 8–24)

   b. The diagnostic wax-up with denture teeth and no labial flange relationship of the residual ridge to the labial of the restoration. The position of the prosthetic teeth is labial to the implant positions. In a traumatic situation, the clinician should always note that teeth, soft tissue, and bone are all lost during a traumatic episode. Augmentation with hard or soft tissue should have been considered prior to uncovering of the implants for this patient. (Fig 8–25)

   c. A four-unit fixed partial denture extending from tooth 7 to tooth 10, supported by two implants and EsthetiCone abutments. (Fig 8–26)

      The restoration emerges through the soft tissue and extends labially due to the lost supporting structures.

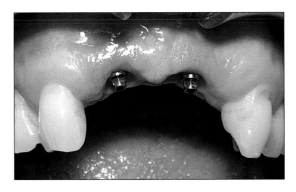

Fig 8-24

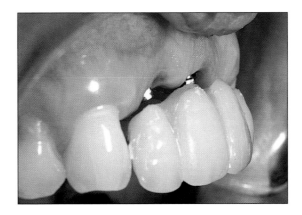

Fig 8-25

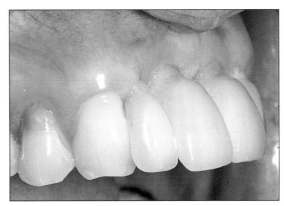

Fig 8-26

Surgery by Dr Donald Hoffman
Laboratory procedure by Toshihiro Takasaki

2. Patient 2

   a. Patient has traumatically lost teeth 9 and 10 and fractured tooth 8. Two osseointegrated implants were placed in position 9 and 10. (Fig 8–27)

   b. Final restoration shows a metal ceramic crown on tooth 8 and a two-unit fixed partial denture on the two implants. EsthetiCone abutments were used for this restoration. Note that the natural tooth and the implants were restored separately. (Fig 8–28)

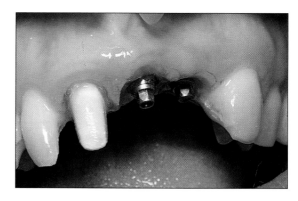

Fig 8-27

Surgery by Dr Richard Martino

Laboratory procedure by Toshihiro Takasaki

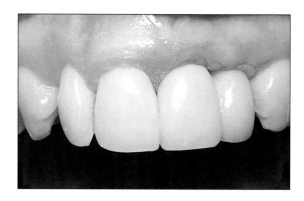

Fig 8-28

References

1. Jemt T. Restoration of osseointegrated implants. Lecture from Chicago Dental Society; Midwinter Meeting, 1992; Chicago, IL.

2. Zarb G, Schmitt A. The longitudinal clinical effectiveness of osseointegrated dental implants in anterior partially edentulous patients. Int J Prosthodont 1993;6: 180–188.

Maxillary Posterior— Partially Edentulous

Goal

1. One implant per tooth replaced
2. Prosthesis independent of natural tooth

Presurgical Needs

1. Mounted diagnostic tests
2. Diagnostic wax-up
3. Surgical guide
4. Radiographic needs
   a. Full mouth periapicals to evaluate prognosis of existing teeth
   b. Panoramic radiograph
   c. Tomogram—to determine vertical height of bone
   d. Computerized axial tomogram—to determine height of bone below the maxillary sinus

Considerations

1. Maxillary sinus position (Fig 9–1)
   a. With inadequate vertical bone height inferior to the maxillary sinus, several options exist including:
      1. No implants
      2. Sinus lift and augmentation
      3. Tuberosity/pterygoid plate implant
      4. Additional surgical procedures
   b. The maxillary sinus often causes the distal implant to incline mesially if the clinician and patient attempt implants with inadequate vertical bone height.[1] (Fig 9–2)

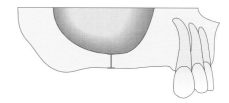

Fig 9-1

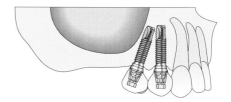

Fig 9-2

2. Buccolingual position[2]

   a. Ideally, the implant should be placed in the center of the anticipated prosthetic tooth. (Fig 9–3)

   b. Following tooth loss in the maxilla, there is vertical bone loss plus buccal width loss. (Fig 9–4)

   c. After tooth loss due to the resorption of alveolar bone, implants placed on the crest of the ridge end up palatal to the center of the anticipated restorative tooth. (Fig 9–5) This should be avoided.

   d. The clinician should attempt to place at least a 4-mm-wide implant. A retrospective study showed that those few implants that fractured were 3.75 mm.[3]

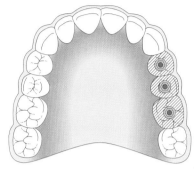

Fig 9-3

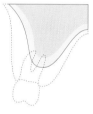

Fig 9-4

9

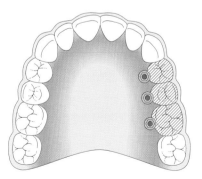

Fig 9-5

e. If significant buccal bone has been lost, an implant placed at the crest of the ridge results in a buccal cantilever. A bending moment is created, which may increase the risk of abutment or fixture fracture,[3] screw joint loosening or fracture of the screw.[4] (Fig 9–6)

1. The goal is to minimize the buccal cantilever in the maxillary posterior region. (Fig 9–7)

f. With poor implant position, sometimes it is necessary to fabricate the fixed partial denture in crossbite with the maxillary buccal cusps occluding in the central groove of the mandibular posterior teeth. (Fig 9–8)

1. Advantages
   a. The force on the implants is directed in the long axis of the implant.
   b. Reduced buccal cantilever.
   c. Reduced bending movement.
2. Disadvantage
   a. Esthetics

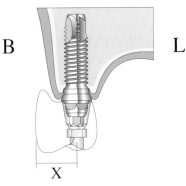

B　　　L

X

Fig 9-6

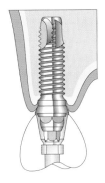

Fig 9-7

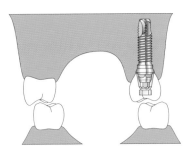

Fig 9-8

3. Angulation problems (Fig 9–9)

   a. Angulation problems are common in the maxillary posterior owing to the contour of the residual bone.

   b. The restorative solution is the angulated abutment or a milled understructure.

   c. However, when the implant is at an angle, prosthesis design should be conservative. Cantilevers to buccal, mesial, and distal result in an increased force on the restoration. The goal is to limit the load on the implant and it components.

   d. The Abutment Selection Kit is helpful in evaluating angulation problems. An impression can be made to the implant or fixture level. A soft-tissue material is used in the region of the implant, and trial abutments can be tried in, in order to select an appropriate one.

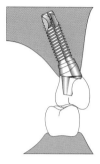

Fig 9–9

4. Number of implants (Fig 9–10)

   a. First, on the lateral cephalometric, CT scan, or panoramic radiograph, determine the potential implant sites. Measure the vertical height of bone below the maxillary sinus. For instance, a minimum of 10 mm vertical height is selected. Then measure the mesiodistal space available for potential implants (from the distal of the anterior tooth bordering the defect to the point where the 10-mm zone of vertical height begins).

If x = mesiodistal space available: then (for 4-mm implants):

If $x \geq 15$ mm, 2 implants are possible.

If $x \geq 22$ mm, 3 implants are possible.

If $x \geq 29$ mm, 4 implants are possible.

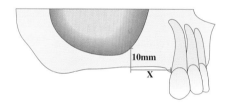

Fig 9-10

9

b. The goal should be at least one implant for each missing posterior tooth to be replaced. Some clinicians suggest one implant per buccal root in the maxillary posterior.

c. Placement of three implants makes the prosthesis more stable. The implant placement can be tripoded, resulting in a more mechanically predictable situation. Screw loosening is less frequent than with a two-implant prosthesis.[4]

5. Cantilevered pontic (Fig 9–11)

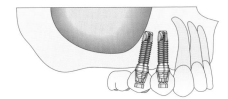

Fig 9-11

a. The clinician should avoid cantilevering a tooth distally, past the last implant.

b. The distal cantilever is a lever arm that increases the load on the components and thus increases the potential for fracture of the abutment screws.[4,5]

c. Disadvantages:

1. Significant masticatory force can be placed on the cantilever if it extends into the molar region.

2. There is a risk of screw fracture or loosening.[4,6]

3. There is risk of implant fracture.[3]

d. Alternatives:

1. Ideally, surgical procedures can be performed to place additional implants.

2. Restoratively, the dentist can simply fabricate the fixed partial denture with one less tooth (without the cantilever).

6. Provisionalization (Fig 9–12)

   a. Some clinicians suggest that provisional-ization is useful in the maxillary posterior.

   b. The provisional restoration can be made of acrylic, which has a low peak impact level.[7] The result is a "shock absorber effect." This allows the implant to be initially loaded at a lower level of force.

   c. It is considered in the maxillary posterior when there is poor bone quality and inadequate quantity.

   d. The clinician may place a provisional to take advantage of the increased cortical-ization of the bone-implant interface that occurs over time.[8] When the definitive restoration is finally placed, the bone implant contact is more mature.

   e. The disadvantage of provisional restorations is fracture and subsequent repair of the provisional. A long-term provisional becomes a high maintenance procedure.

   f. A provisional made of methyl-methacry-late is flexible, and this flexibility may place adverse stresses on the implants. Provisional restorations are thus less effective than metal frameworks, and some clinicians use them for a short period of time or not at all.

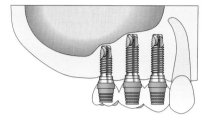

Fig 9-12

9

Patient Examples[4,9-11]

The following patient examples are intended to assist the restorative dentist in planning optimal implant placement. For some of the clinical situations several treatment options and the anticipated advantages and disadvantages are suggested. These are intended as guidelines only and the clinician must remember that each patient is unique with specific restorative requirements.

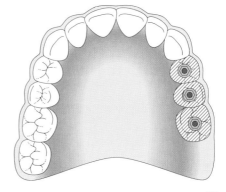

Fig 9-13

▼ Missing: All Maxillary Left Posterior Teeth (Fig 9–13)

1. Considerations
   a. Size of maxillary sinus and vertical height of bone below it (need 10 mm)
   b. Vertical space from ridge to opposing occlusion
   c. Posterior extent of opposing occlusion
   d. Width of crestal bone (6 mm) needed
2. Plan
   a. The goal is one implant per missing tooth.
   b. Often implants are possible only to the first molar region, owing to the presence of the maxillary sinus. (Fig 9–14)

      The clinician is forced to accept an occlusal plane that extends to the first molar region. The result is no replacement of the maxillary second molar.
   c. Three implants and a three-unit fixed partial denture or four implants and a four-unit fixed partial denture.
   d. No posterior cantilevers.

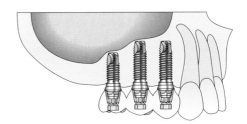

Fig 9-14

▼ Missing: Maxillary Left Premolars and First Molar

1. Considerations
   a. Vertical height of bone needed inferior to the maxillary sinus (10 mm)
   b. Vertical space from the ridge to the opposing occlusion
   c. Width of bone (6 mm) needed
   d. Opposing occlusion and the number of teeth that will require centric contacts from the proposed implant fixed partial denture

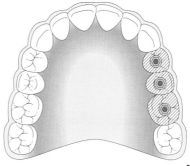

Fig 9-15

2. Plan
   a. The goal is one implant per missing tooth. (Fig 9–15)
   b. Three implants and a three-unit fixed partial denture should be placed.
   c. Two implants and a three-unit partial denture (Fig 9–16) should be avoided because the cantilever places increased bending on the restoration and an increased chance of abutment screw fracture.[4]

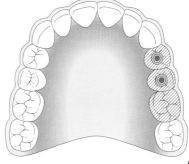

Fig 9-16

9

▼ Missing: Maxillary Left Premolars

1. Considerations
    a. The vertical height of space to opposing dentition should be measured intraorally or on diagnostic casts.
    b. The maxillary sinus in the second premolar region is often enlarged. (10 mm of vertical bone height is needed.)
    c. The buccolingual width of the alveolar ridge should be measured (6 mm is needed).
    d. The root inclination of neighboring natural teeth should be evaluated on radiographs. Sometimes the angulation of the roots is such that it hinders implant placement.

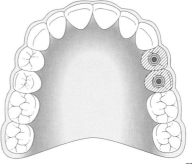

Fig 9-17

2. Plan
    a. The goal is a two-unit fixed partial denture with one implant per missing tooth. (Fig 9–17)

3. Alternate plan (Fig 9–18)
    a. One implant can be placed in the first premolar region and a pontic used to replace the second premolar. The pontic can be connected to the natural tooth abutment (molar) with a rigid or nonrigid attachment. This option should be avoided.
    b. Disadvantages:
        1. Connecting to the natural tooth creates a problem due to the difference in mobility between a tooth and an implant (see partially edentulous considerations, Chapter 7).
        2. This option has a high risk of mechanical problems.

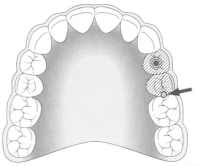

Fig 9-18

▼ Missing: Maxillary Left Premolars, Molars, Canine and Lateral Incisor (Fig 9–19)

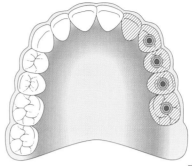

Fig 9-19

1. Considerations
   a. Often there is a labial concavity due to bone loss in the lateral incisor and cuspid area. (6 mm ridge width is needed.)
   b. The size of the maxillary sinus and vertical height of bone inferior to it should be noted. (10 mm is needed.)
   c. The occlusal scheme must be planned prior to implant placement. With a missing canine and lateral incisor, natural canine disclusion is not possible.
   d. Vertical space available.

2. Plan
   a. The goal is one implant per missing posterior tooth restored; and as many implants as possible.
   b. Avoid posterior cantilevers.
   c. Occlusion: consider group function with multiple contacts on the partial denture in lateral excursion.
   d. Surgical augmentation of the cuspid and lateral incisor site should be considered.

9

Patient Presentations

1. Patient 1

   a. Teeth 2, 3, and 4 have been lost and three osseointegrated implants with Estheti-Cone abutments have been placed in position. Please note that three implants were used in order to replace the three natural teeth. (Fig 9–20)

   b. The definitive restoration is a three-unit fixed partial denture. The occlusal view of the restoration shows screw access holes in the metal occlusals. The width of the occlusal surface (buccolingual) is slightly reduced when compared to normal molar size. Metal occlusals were used because the opposing dentition in the mandibular arch was previously restored with metal occlusals. (Fig 9–21)

   c. Facial view of the restoration shown in place. Note that this is a three-unit fixed partial denture. The splinted crowns transfer the stress between the three implants and components upon loading. (Fig 9–22)

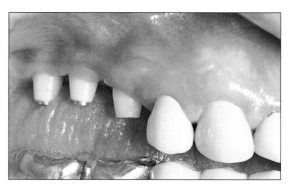

Fig 9-20

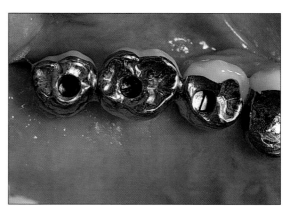

Fig 9-21

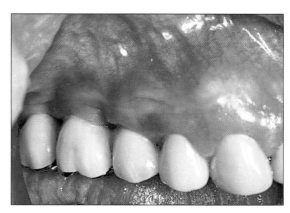

Fig 9-22

Surgery by Dr Peter Moy
Laboratory procedures by Gary Nunakawa

2. Patient 2

   a. Teeth 12, 13, 14, and 15 are missing. Three osseointegrated implants were placed for a more predictable restoration as compared to two implants. The three implants were placed in the maxillary posterior region with EsthetiCone abutments. (Fig 9–23)

   b. The definitive restoration is a three-unit fixed partial denture. Note that no cantilevers were placed distally to add another tooth. If this is done, excessive forces and a bending movement are created around the restoration, and the result is more frequent fractures of the abutment screws. If an additional tooth is needed by the patient or for occlusal stability, an additional implant should be placed in this area. (Fig 9–24)

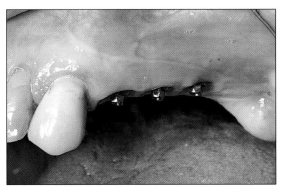

Fig 9-23

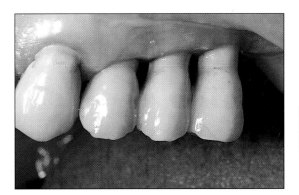

Fig 9-24

Surgery by Dr Neil Hagen
Laboratory procedures by Toshihiro Takasaki

3. Patient 3

   a. Due to the presence of the maxillary sinus, only two osseointegrated implants were placed in tooth positions 12 and 13. The patient refused augmentation procedures that were offered, so only two implants were possible. (Fig 9–25)

   b. The definitive restoration is a two-unit fixed partial denture in place with no cantilevers distally. If a cantilever is placed on this restoration it would result in a more unstable restoration with possible fracture or loosening of the components. (Fig 9–26)

   c. Two-unit fixed partial denture on two osseointegrated implants. (Fig 9–27)

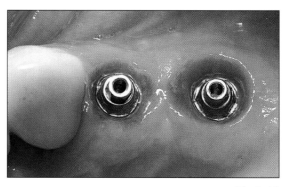

Fig 9-25

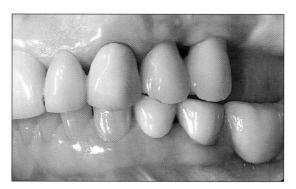

Fig 9-26

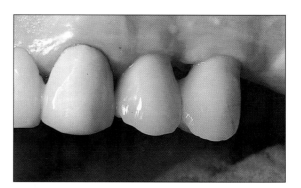

Fig 9-27

Surgery by Dr Richard Marinello
Laboratory procedures by Toshihiro Takasaki

References

1. Jemt T. Restoration of osseointegrated implants. Lecture for Chicago Dental Society; Midwinter Meeting, 1992; Chicago, IL.

2. Rangert B, Jemt T, Jorneus L. Forces and moments on Brånemark implants. Int J Oral Maxillofac Implants 1989;4:241–247.

3. Rangert B, Krogh P, Langer B. Bending overload and implant fracture: A retrospective clinical analysis. Int J Oral Maxillofac Implants 1995;10:326–334.

4. Jemt T, Lekholm U. Oral implant treatment in posterior partially edentulous jaws: a 5-year follow-up report. Int J Oral Maxillofac Implants 1993;8:635–640.

5. Rangert B, Sullivan R. Learning from history: The transition from full arch to posterior partial restorations. Nobelpharma News 1995;9:6–7.

6. Lekholm U, van Steenberghe D, Herrmann I. Osseointegrated implants in the treatment of posterior partially edentulous jaws: A 5-year multi-center study. Int J Oral Maxillofac Implants 1994;9:627–635.

7. Skalak R. Biomedical considerations in osseointegrated prosthesis. J Prosthet Dent 1983;49:843–848.

8. Carlsson GE, Haraldson T. Functional response. In: Brånemark PI, Zarb G, Albrektsson T, eds. Tissue-integrated Prostheses: Osseointegration in Clinical Dentistry. Chicago: Quintessence; 1985:155–163.

9. Bahat O. Treatment planning and placement of implants in the posterior maxillae: Report of 732 consecutive Nobelpharma implants. Int J Oral Maxillofac Implants 1993;8:151–161.

10. Bahat O. Osseointegrated implants in the maxillary tuberosity: Report on 45 consecutive patients. Int J Oral Maxillofac Implants 1992;7:459–467.

11. Zarb G, Schmitt A. The longitudinal clinical effectiveness of osseointegrated dental implants in posterior partially edentulous patients. Int J Prosthodont 1993;6:189–196.

9

Mandibular Anterior—Partially Edentulous

Goal

1. Fixed prosthesis
2. Esthetics less critical (than in the maxillary anterior) for most patients

Presurgical Needs

1. Mounted diagnostic casts
2. Diagnostic wax-up
3. Surgical guide
4. Examination of smile line

   Measure the distance from lower lip to the crest of residual ridge. Some patient's mandibular ridges are visible when the patient smiles or speaks, resulting in high esthetic requirements. This should be done especially for patients with recent extractions.

5. Radiographic needs
   a. Full mouth periapicals to evaluate prognosis of existing dentition
   b. Panoramic radiograph
   c. Tomogram: rarely needed
   d. Computerized axial tomogram: rarely needed

Considerations

1. Ridge width

   a. In the mandibular anterior region, the residual ridge is often narrow (Fig 10–1), normally with a labiolingual width less than the 6 mm needed to accommodate a 4-mm implant.

   b. One option is reduction of the ridge height (Fig 10–2) and placement of implants at a more inferior position. In some patients with an abundance of vertical bone height and a low lower lip line, this option may be desirable. The clinician must consider the amount of reduction needed and how it will affect the long-term prognosis of neighboring teeth.

   c. Reduction of the height (Fig 10–3) can be achieved because there is usually more than adequate vertical bone height in the mandibular anterior region of partially edentulous patients.

   d. A second option is to augment the ridge width and place implants. This is rarely necessary except in instances of severe trauma or surgical defect.

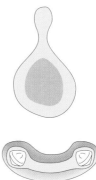

Fig 10-1

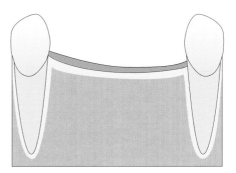

Fig 10-2

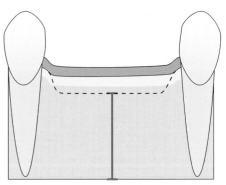

Fig 10-3

2. Mesiodistal width of incisors (Fig 10–4)

  a. Mandibular incisors are narrow (4 to 5 mm) mesiodistally. It is impossible to place one implant per tooth.

    Where x = mesiodistal space available:

    If $x > 7$ mm, 1 implant is possible.

    If $x \geq 15$ mm, 2 implants are possible.

    If $x \geq 22$ mm, 3 implants are possible.

3. Vertical height of defect (Fig 10–5)

  a. When mandibular incisors are lost, there sometimes is a significant loss of vertical bone height. The result is a significant difference in ridge height between the edentulous space and the dentulous segments. The prosthesis is often best made with denture teeth and denture acrylic on a metal framework to simulate the lost gingiva.

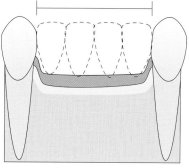

Fig 10-4

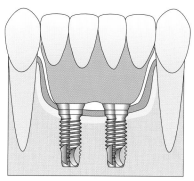

Fig 10-5

10

Patient Examples[1]

The following patient examples are intended to assist the restorative dentist in planning optimal implant placement. For some of the clinical situations several treatment options and the anticipated advantages and disadvantages are suggested. These are intended as guidelines only, and the clinician must remember that each patient is unique with specific restorative requirements.

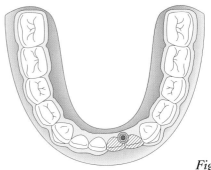

Fig 10-6

▼ Missing: Mandibular Left-Lateral and Left-Central Incisors

1. Considerations
   a. Labiolingual ridge width (6 mm needed)
   b. Mesiodistal space available
   c. Vertical space available
2. Plan (Fig 10–6)
   a. When two mandibular incisors are missing, one implant retaining a two-tooth fixed partial denture can be planned. The implant may be restored as a single-implant restoration, with the restoration shaped to simulate two teeth.
   b. When two incisors are missing, the mesiodistal distance is often significantly less than 14 mm. In this instance, only one implant is possible.
3. Disadvantage
   a. A see-saw effect has been created over the single implant. (Fig 10–7) This may cause a bending movement and loosen the screw. If space is too wide this is not a predictable restoration. This occurs infrequently because less force occurs here than in the posterior region.

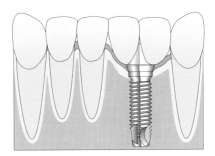

Fig 10-7

▼ Missing: Mandibular Central Incisors and Left-Lateral Incisor

1. Considerations
   a. Mesiodistal space available
   b. Labiolingual ridge width (6 mm needed)
   c. Vertical space available
2. Plan (Fig 10–8)
   a. Two implants if mesiodistal width ≥ 15 mm.
   b. Three-unit fixed partial denture on two implants.

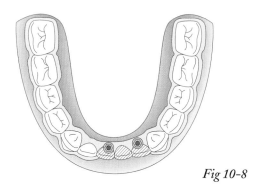

Fig 10-8

▼ Missing: All Mandibular Incisors

1. Considerations
   a. Labiolingual ridge width (6 mm needed)
   b. Mesiodistal space available
   c. Vertical space available
2. Plan (Fig 10–9)
   a. Two implants if $x \geq 15$ mm.
      1. A four-unit fixed partial denture can be fabricated on only two implants because relatively little force is placed in this region during function.
   b. Three implants if $x \geq 22$ mm.

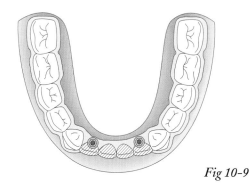

Fig 10-9

10

▼ Missing: All Mandibular Incisors and Right Canine

1. Considerations
   a. Labiolingual ridge width (6 mm needed)
   b. Mesiodistal space available (x)
   c. Vertical space available
2. Plan (Fig 10–10)
   a. Two implants if 15 mm $\leq$ x < 22 mm.
      Three implants if x $\geq$ 22 mm.
   b. Five-unit fixed partial denture.
   c. The occlusion must be carefully evaluated prior to implant placement. An occlusal scheme should be established with contacts on multiple prosthetic teeth and simultaneous contacts on natural teeth if possible.

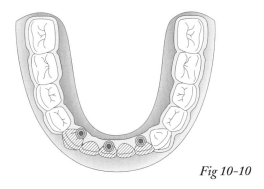

Fig 10-10

▼ Missing: All Mandibular Incisors and Canines

1. Considerations
   a. Labiolingual ridge width
   b. Mesiodistal space (x)
   c. Vertical space available
2. Plan (Fig 10–11)
   a. Three implants if 22 mm $\leq$ x < 29 mm.
      Four implants if x $\geq$ 29 mm.
   b. Strive to have implant within the body of the anticipated prosthetic tooth. Avoid interproximal placement as esthetics are often compromised.
   c. The occlusal scheme should be with multiple contacts on natural and prosthetic teeth.

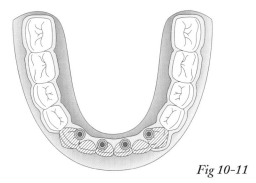

Fig 10-11

Patient Presentations

1. Patient 1
   a. The patient has lost teeth 20 to 26. The treatment plan includes a hip graft and placement of four osseointegrated implants. The hip graft was placed and allowed to heal and the implants placed at a second procedure. (Fig 10–12)

   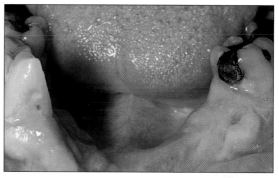

   Fig 10-12

   b. Definitive restoration in place shows four osseointegrated implants supported the seven-unit fixed partial denture. This restoration is very similar to the fixed detachable prosthesis for the completely edentulous patient. This design is very useful for patients who have lost teeth and large portions of the mandibular alveolar ridge. (Fig 10–13)

   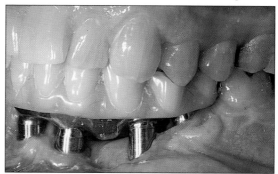

   Fig 10-13

   c. The restoration allows easy access for hygiene. (Fig 10–14)
   d. A normal esthetic result is achieved with denture teeth, acrylic, and metal framework. (Fig 10–15)

   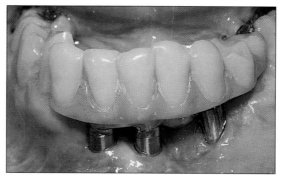

   Fig 10-14

10

   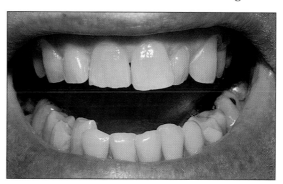

Surgery by Dr Michael Stohle
Laboratory procedures by Steve Stevens

Fig 10-15

2. Patient 2

   a. Only teeth 21, 22, 26, and 27 remain in the mandibular arch. Two osseointegrated implants were placed in tooth position 23 and 26. (Fig 10–16)

   b. Implants were uncovered and standard abutments were positioned while the tissue was allowed to heal. (Fig 10–17)

   c. The definitive restoration is a four-unit fixed partial denture supported by osseointegrated implants. One implant per missing tooth is not necessary, because this is an anterior restoration; it is not possible, owing to inadequate mesiodistal space. This restoration extended directly to the fixtures with no abutments in between. (Fig 10–18)

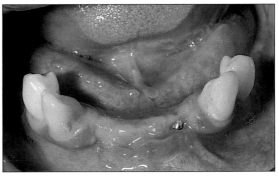

Fig 10-16

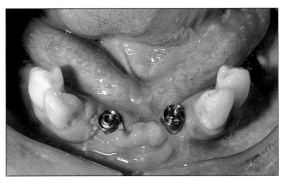

Fig 10-17

Surgery by Dr Peter Moy
Laboratory procedures by Wynn Hornberg

Reference

1. Zarb G, Schmitt A. The longitudinal clinical effectiveness of osseointegrated dental implants in anterior partially edentulous patients. Int J Prosthodont 1993;6:180–188.

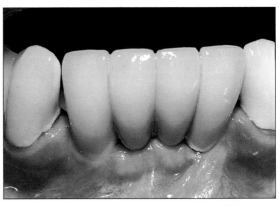

Fig 10-18

Mandibular Posterior—Partially Edentulous

Goal

1. Prosthesis with no connection to natural tooth
2. A minimum of one implant per missing tooth
   (Note: Some clinicians suggest one implant per missing root.)

Presurgical Needs

1. Mounted diagnostic casts
2. Diagnostic wax-up
3. Surgical guide
4. Radiographic needs
   a. Full-mouth periapicals to evaluate prognosis of remaining natural teeth
   b. Panoramic radiograph
   c. Tomogram: often needed to determine vertical height of bone above the inferior alveolar nerve
   d. Computerized axial tomogram: to determine vertical height of bone above the inferior alveolar nerve

Considerations

1. Ridge width (Fig 11–1)

   a. Buccolingual width of ridge must be measured. The ridge is often too narrow to accommodate a 4-mm implant. The dentist should place 4-mm or wider implants for the mandibular posterior in order to reduce the incidence of implant fracture. A clinical retrospective study showed fractures occurring only with 3.75-mm implants.[1]

   b. Surgical solutions for narrow ridge:

      1. Ridge height can be surgically reduced until the ridge width is adequate for implant placement. However, the height above the alveolar nerve is the limiting factor. Height reduction is not always possible.

      2. Augmentation will solve the problem of inadequate ridge width. Augmentation can be done simultaneous to implant placement or as a separate procedure.

      3. The ridge may be split at the crest and augmented. The region is allowed to heal and then implants can be placed.

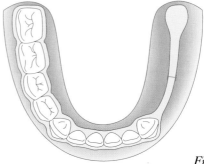

Fig 11-1

2. Supereruption of opposing occlusion (Fig 11–2)

a. The occlusal plane must be evaluated with mounted diagnostic casts. When teeth have been missing for several years, the vertical space between the arches is often reduced. The maxillary teeth may be touching the mandibular ridge.

b. If the vertical space is too small to fit components, there are several options:

1. Minor enameloplasty or occlusal adjustment of the opposing dentition
2. Restoration of the opposing (maxillary) arch
3. Orthodontics
4. A segmental osteotomy

This procedure can surgically reposition the malpositioned maxillary posterior teeth. Orthodontics, combined with the osteotomy, will improve the final result by providing additional vertical space and correcting the irregular plane of occlusion.

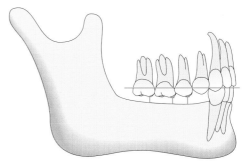

Fig 11-2

3. Mesiodistal width of edentulous space[2,3] (Fig 11–3)

a. There may be inadequate vertical height of bone above the mental nerve and an edentulous space extending distal to the cuspid. The region should be considered in two segments: anterior and posterior to the mental foramen and loop.

b. Measure the distance from the most distal tooth to the anterior loop of the mental nerve.

c. Measure from the mental foramen distal until the vertical height limitation above is reached. The vertical height limitation is the length of the shortest implant considered acceptable for this patient. Some clinicians select 10 mm as the shortest desired implant.

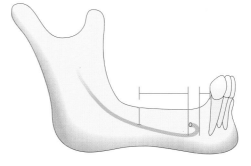

Fig 11-3

11

4. Inadequate vertical height of bone

   If vertical height above inferior alveolar is less than needed (Fig 11–4), options include:

   a. A wider (5 mm) and shorter implant.

   b. The ridge can be augmented.

   c. The inferior alveolar can be laterally repositioned and implants placed. The surgeon is encouraged to consider the risks and benefits thoroughly.

5. Cantilever (Fig 11–5)

   a. An implant in the mandibular first premolar region is often not possible due to the position of the mental nerve. The restorative dentist may extend a pontic into this area if three implants are in the molar region. This cantilever places additional stress on the implant and implant components, but some clinicians accept this option because of the lower occlusal demands in the first premolar region compared to molars.

   b. A posterior cantilever in the molar region should be avoided. The result would be a higher incident of abutment screw and implant fracture.[1,4]

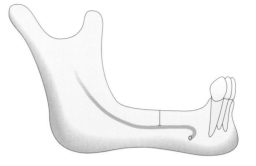

Fig 11-4

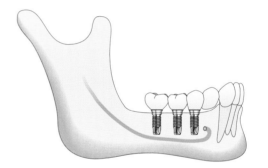

Fig 11-5

6. Cross-sectional contour of posterior mandible

   a. There is a lingual concavity in the mandibular molar region that makes vertical implants difficult for some patients. (Fig 11–6)

   b. Some ridges exhibit a buccal concavity just below the crest of the ridge. (Fig 11–7)

   Surgical augmentation is often necessary prior to implant placement. (Fig 11–8)

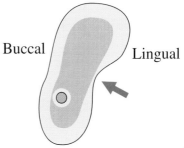

Fig 11-6

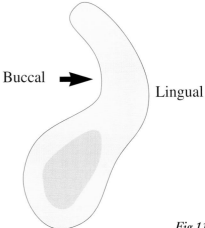

Fig 11-7

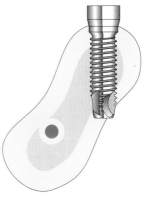

Fig 11-8

11

Patient Examples[4,5]

The following patient examples are intended to assist the restorative dentist in planning optimal implant placement. For some of the clinical situations several treatment options are given, along with advantages and disadvantages. These are intended as guidelines only and the clinician must remember that each patient is unique with specific restorative requirements.

▼ Missing: Mandibular Right First and Second Molars (Fig 11–9)

1. Considerations
   a. Height of bone above inferior alveolar nerve (10 mm needed)
   b. Labiolingual width of bone (6 mm needed)
   c. Mesiodistal space available
   d. Vertical space available
2. Plan
   a. Two implants and two-unit fixed partial denture can be placed. The problem with placing only two implants is that they are in a straight line. This option has more frequent screw loosening, abutment screw fracture, and implant fracture than does a three-implant restoration.[5,6]
   b. Three implants can be placed for some patients. The advantage is less frequent screw loosening.[1,5,6]

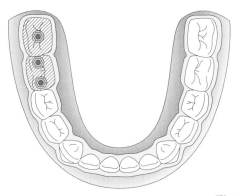

Fig 11-9

▼ Missing: Mandibular Right Molars and Second Premolar

1. Considerations
   a. Height of bone above inferior alveolar nerve (10 mm needed)
   b. Labiolingual width of bone (6 mm needed)
   c. Mesiodistal space available
   d. Mental foramen and mental nerve position
   e. Vertical space available
2. Plan
   a. The goal is one implant per tooth. Three implants and a three-unit fixed partial denture should be placed. (Fig 11–10)
3. Alternate Plans
   a. A three-unit fixed partial denture with two implants and a cantilever over the second premolar locations should be avoided. This places an increased load on the implant components. (Fig 11–11)
   b. A three-unit fixed partial denture with two implants and a pontic for the first molar should be avoided. Usually if two implants can be placed in these positions, there is adequate bone for a third implant. The ideal solution is one implant per missing tooth. (Fig 11–12)

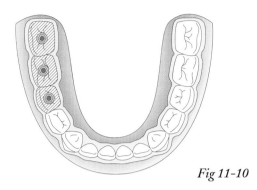

Fig 11-10

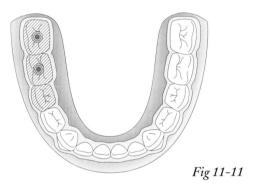

Fig 11-11

11

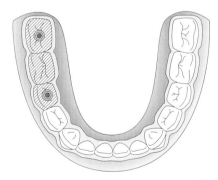

Fig 11-12

▼ Missing: Mandibular Right Molars and Premolars (Fig 11–13)

1. Considerations
   a. Height of bone above inferior alveolar nerve (10 mm needed)
   b. Labiolingual width of bone (6 mm needed)
   c. Mesiodistal space available
   d. Position of the mental nerve
      1. The space anterior and posterior to the mental foramen and loop should be considered as two separate segments.
   e. Vertical space available
2. Plan
   a. The goal is one implant per missing tooth. Three or four implants should be planned depending on the space available.
   b. A four-unit fixed partial denture can be planned if three or four implants are placed. Three implants can be placed in the molar and second premolar position. A four-unit fixed partial denture with a cantilever in the first premolar can be placed on the three implants.
   c. Ideally, a four-unit fixed partial denture should be supported by four implants. (Fig 11–14)

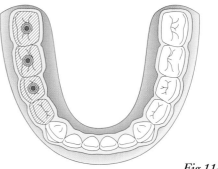

Fig 11-13

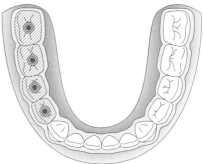

Fig 11-14

▼ Missing: Mandibular Right First and Second Molars and First Premolar (Fig 11–15)

1. Considerations
   a. Prognosis of the mandibular right second premolar (natural tooth)
   b. Position of the mental nerve and canal (which may prevent use of the first premolar space for implant placement)
   c. Position of the inferior alveolar nerve
   d. Vertical space available
2. Plan
   a. A three-unit fixed partial denture can be placed, from the canine to the second premolar, with natural tooth abutments. Two or three implants and a two-unit fixed partial denture restore the missing molars. (Fig 11–16) The implant restoration and the natural tooth–supported restoration are separate.
   b. (Fig 11–17) A single-implant restoration can be placed for the first premolar and the molars replaced with two or three implants and a two-unit fixed partial denture. The weak link of this plan is the natural second premolar. If it fails, both restorations must be remade into a four-unit fixed partial denture on the three implants. A more predictable restoration may be made without the natural second premolar.
   c. (Fig 11–18) The second premolar can be removed if it has a poor prognosis. Ideally, four implants are placed and a four-unit fixed partial denture fabricated replacing the premolars and the molars.

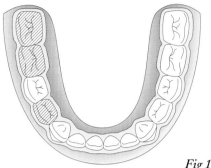

Fig 11-15

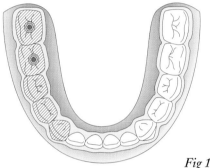

Fig 11-16

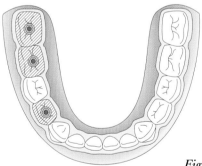

Fig 11-17

11

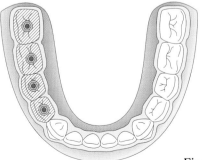

Fig 11-18

Patient Presentations

1. Patient 1

    a. The patient has lost teeth 18 and 19, and teeth 14 and 15 have extruded. Composite and orthodontic wire are used to prevent further supereruption of 14 and 15. Three osseointegrated implants have been placed in the position of 18 and 19. (Fig 11–19)

    b. With three osseointegrated implants, the load is distributed over more implants. The three implants are slightly tripoded, which more optimally distributes the stress and reduces the chance of overload. This results in a more stable restoration with less frequent loosening and fracturing of gold screws. (Fig 11–20)

    c. Facial view of the restoration supported by three osseointegrated implants. (Fig 11–21)

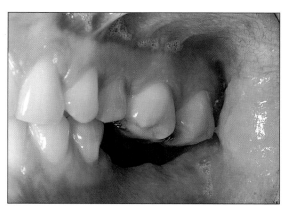

Fig 11-19

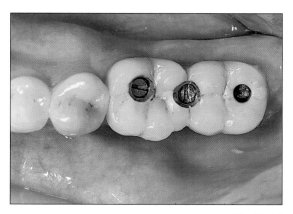

Fig 11-20

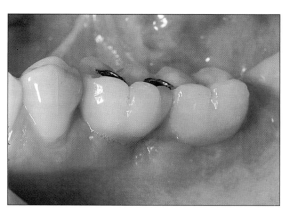

Fig 11-21

Surgery by Dr Michael Stohle

Laboratory procedures by Toshihiro Takasaki

2. Patient 2

   a. Occlusal view of patient who has teeth 29, 30, and 31 missing. Three osseointegrated implants, along with EsthetiCone abutments, have been placed. (Fig 11–22)

   b. Facial view of the metal ceramic restoration shows a three-unit fixed partial denture on the three implants. Tooth 28 has been restored with a metal ceramic crown separate from the implant restoration. (Fig 11–23)

   c. Occlusal view of the same restoration showing three implants retaining a three-unit fixed partial denture and a single crown on tooth 28, the natural tooth. (Fig 11–24)

Surgery by Dr Peter Chemello
Laboratory procedures by Toshihiro Takasaki

References

1. Rangert B, Krogh P, Langer B. Bending overload and implant fracture: A retrospective clinical analysis. Int J Oral Maxillofac Implants 1995;10:326–334.

2. Jemt T. Restoration of osseointegrated implants. Lecture for Chicago Dental Society; Midwinter Meeting, 1992: Chicago, IL.

3. Hobo S, Ichida E, Garcia L. Osseointegration and Occlusal Rehabilitation. Tokyo: Quintessence; 1991:55–86.

4. Zarb G, Schmitt A. The longitudinal clinical effectiveness of osseointegrated dental implants in posterior partially edentulous patients. Int J Prosthodont 1993;6:189–196.

5. Jemt T, Lekholm U. Oral implant treatment in posterior partially edentulous jaws: A 5-year follow-up report. Int J Oral Maxillofac Implants 1993;8:635–640.

6. Lekholm U, van Steenberghe D, Herrmann I. Osseointegrated implants in the treatment of posterior partially edentulous jaws: A 5-year multi-center study. Int J Oral Maxillofac Implants 1994;9:627–635.

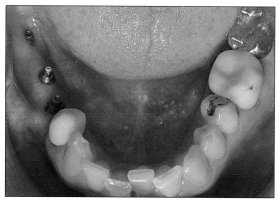

Fig 11-22

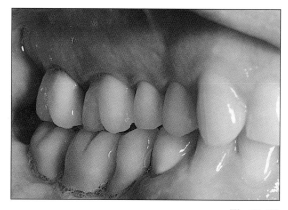

Fig 11-23

11

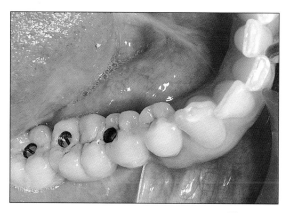

Fig 11-24

12

Sequencing Flowsheets

Information collecting for treatment planning of restorative dental patients is a very critical step in decision making. The following sequence flow sheets provide an outline that the restorative dentist can follow when evaluating partially edentulous and completely edentulous patients. Included are normal categories of the medical history review, external and intraoral examination. Careful attention should be paid to mounted diagnostic casts. The restorative dentist should examine them for anatomical structures, vertical space, ridge width, and maxillo-mandibular relations. As with most patients radiographic analysis is also crucial for implant patients. The restorative dentist should carefully evaluate the available vertical height of bone and ridge width. The number of implants necessary to complete a successful restoration and the position in placement of those implants should also be considered.

Preliminary Data

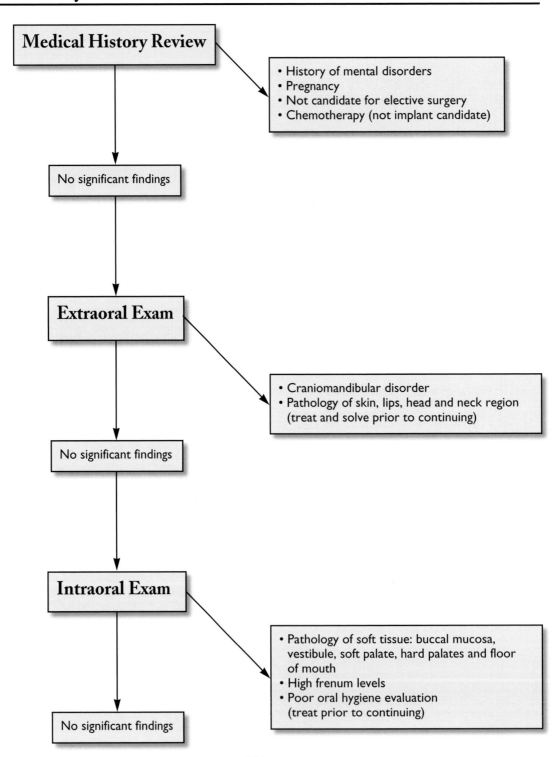

Medical History Review

• History of mental disorders
• Pregnancy
• Not candidate for elective surgery
• Chemotherapy (not implant candidate)

No significant findings

Extraoral Exam

• Craniomandibular disorder
• Pathology of skin, lips, head and neck region
  (treat and solve prior to continuing)

No significant findings

Intraoral Exam

• Pathology of soft tissue: buccal mucosa,
  vestibule, soft palate, hard palates and floor
  of mouth
• High frenum levels
• Poor oral hygiene evaluation
  (treat prior to continuing)

No significant findings

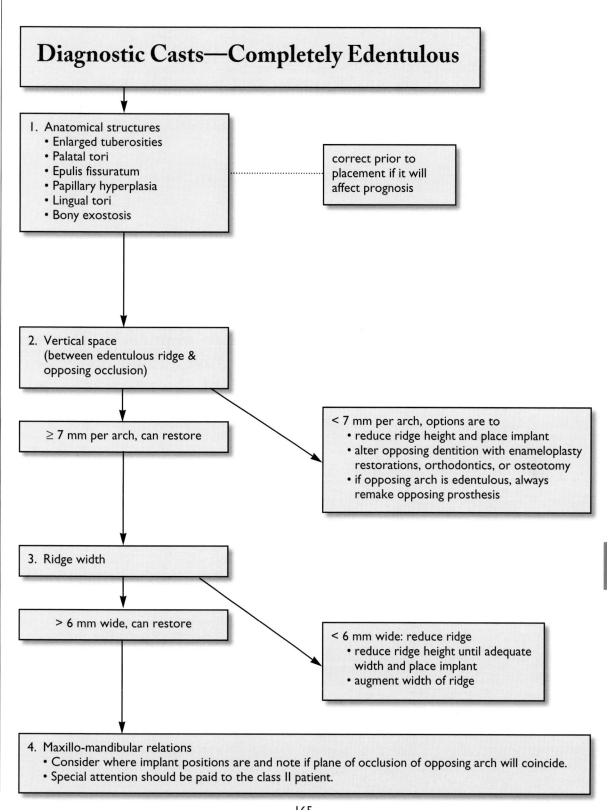

Diagnostic Casts—Completely Edentulous

1. Anatomical structures
   • Enlarged tuberosities
   • Palatal tori
   • Epulis fissuratum
   • Papillary hyperplasia
   • Lingual tori
   • Bony exostosis

correct prior to placement if it will affect prognosis

2. Vertical space
   (between edentulous ridge & opposing occlusion)

≥ 7 mm per arch, can restore

< 7 mm per arch, options are to
• reduce ridge height and place implant
• alter opposing dentition with enameloplasty restorations, orthodontics, or osteotomy
• if opposing arch is edentulous, always remake opposing prosthesis

3. Ridge width

> 6 mm wide, can restore

< 6 mm wide: reduce ridge
• reduce ridge height until adequate width and place implant
• augment width of ridge

4. Maxillo-mandibular relations
   • Consider where implant positions are and note if plane of occlusion of opposing arch will coincide.
   • Special attention should be paid to the class II patient.

12

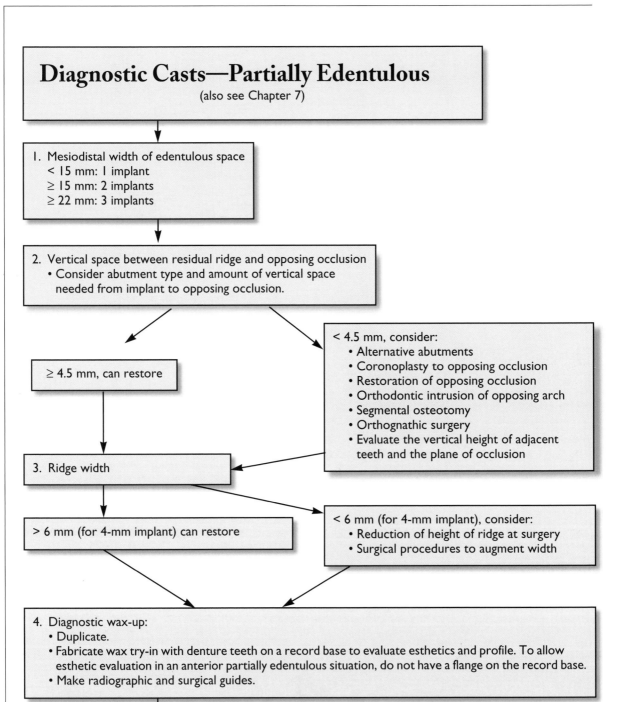

Diagnostic Casts—Partially Edentulous
(also see Chapter 7)

1. Mesiodistal width of edentulous space
   < 15 mm: 1 implant
   ≥ 15 mm: 2 implants
   ≥ 22 mm: 3 implants

2. Vertical space between residual ridge and opposing occlusion
   • Consider abutment type and amount of vertical space needed from implant to opposing occlusion.

≥ 4.5 mm, can restore

< 4.5 mm, consider:
   • Alternative abutments
   • Coronoplasty to opposing occlusion
   • Restoration of opposing occlusion
   • Orthodontic intrusion of opposing arch
   • Segmental osteotomy
   • Orthognathic surgery
   • Evaluate the vertical height of adjacent teeth and the plane of occlusion

3. Ridge width

> 6 mm (for 4-mm implant) can restore

< 6 mm (for 4-mm implant), consider:
   • Reduction of height of ridge at surgery
   • Surgical procedures to augment width

4. Diagnostic wax-up:
   • Duplicate.
   • Fabricate wax try-in with denture teeth on a record base to evaluate esthetics and profile. To allow esthetic evaluation in an anterior partially edentulous situation, do not have a flange on the record base.
   • Make radiographic and surgical guides.

5. Radiographic analysis
   • Note pathologies, radiolucencies, and radiopacities: treat prior to treatment.
   • Note quality of bone, thickness of cortical bone, density of medullary bone, and vertical height of alveolar bone in anticipated implant sites.
   • Implant lengths are 7–20 mm. Many clinicians consider 10 mm the minimum vertical height.

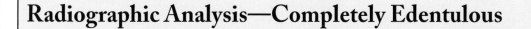

Radiographic Analysis—Completely Edentulous

1. Vertical height of available bone (panoramic or lateral cephalometric radiograph)

> 10 mm

< 10 mm, consider:
   a. Short, wide implant
   b. Augmentation of ridge

2. Mesiodistal space (panoramic radiograph)
   • Mandible
     Identify mental foramen

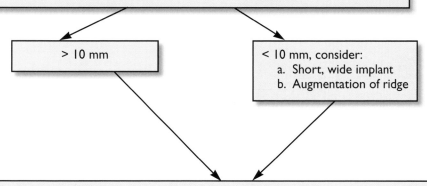

• Maxilla
  Identify incisive canal and maxillary sinuses

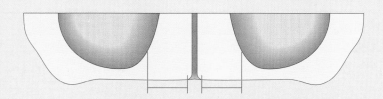

Note the height of bone available and mark where the minimum vertical height of bone ends.
Measure the mesiodistal space where adequate vertical height of bone is available.
If there is inadequate bone for implants, augmentation may be necessary.

12

Radiographic Analysis—Partially Edentulous

1. Vertical height of anticipated site (via periapical, panoramic, or lateral cephalometric radiograph; tomogram, CT)

> 10 mm, can restore

< 10 mm, mandibular surgical options include:
  a. Surgical procedures:
    1. Augment ridge
    2. Reposition the inferior alveolar nerve
    3. Shorter, wider implant
    4. No implant

maxillary options:
  advanced surgical procedures include:
    1. Sinus lift
    2. Augmentation
    3. Bone grafting

2. Mesiodistal space (via panoramic radiograph, lateral cephalometric)
  Identify region of adequate vertical height of bone, then measure mesiodistal space (x).

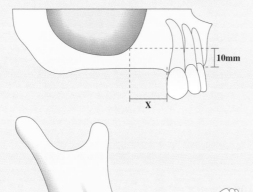

10mm

x

- Maxilla
  For 4-mm implant:
  x < 15 mm = 1 implant
  x ≥ 15 mm = 2 implants
  x ≥ 22 mm = 3 implants

- Mandible (panoramic or lateral radiograph)
  For 4-mm implant:
  x < 15 mm = 1 implant
  x ≥ 15 mm = 2 implants
  x ≥ 22 mm = 3 implants

Consider mandible in 2 segments, anterior and posterior to the loop of the mental nerve.

Occlusion

A philosophy of occlusion is a very elusive goal for conventional and implant restorative dentistry. There is no single concept of occlusion that can be applied to all patients. The unique patient situation must be evaluated by the clinician. The factors that must be considered include: load, opposing occlusion, opposing restorative material, parafunctional habits, existing occlusal scheme, plane of occlusion, interarch distance, and dental history. The following occlusal discussion is divided into four categories: single-tooth restoration, partially edentulous restoration, completely edentulous restoration, and combination of completely and partially edentulous restorations. These are intended as guidelines only and the clinician must remember that each patient is unique with specific restorative requirements.

Single Tooth Restoration

1. Centric contact of the single-tooth implant restoration should be lighter in casual intercuspation and equal to the natural teeth in maximum intercuspation. (Fig 13–1)

   Some clinicians will reduce the size of contact in an attempt to compensate for the lack of a periodontal ligament around the implant. If the implant restoration is taken out of occlusion the risk is super-eruption of the opposing dentition.

2. The implant crown should avoid contact in excursive movements if possible. This is especially true for posterior teeth.

3. In some excursive movements, contact may occur on an implant-supported single tooth. (Fig 13–2)

   An attempt should be made to share the load simultaneously with the natural teeth. This often occurs with anterior replacement, especially with canines.

4. For molars, some clinicians suggest making the occlusal surface smaller buccolingually to prevent eccentric contacts to the restorative complex. (Fig 13–3)

   The clinician should note the mesiodistal space to be restored, prior to implant placement. If this space is wider than a single molar, caution should be exercised. Some clinicians will prefer a three-unit fixed partial denture over an implant-supported molar because of the risk of screw loosening, dissolution of cement in the crown, or implant fracture.

5. For the single-tooth replacement, the weak link of the system is often the screw joint. If the system is overloaded the screw joint is loosened.

6. Because of the high occlusal demands for single missing molars, some clinicians will plan two implants. These implants are splinted together by a single restoration (a two-unit fixed partial denture). (Fig 13–4)

7. The occlusal contact on the single implant crown should be centered over the implant. If the contact is on the lingual or buccal cusp far from the implant, a bending force will result. This will increase the possibility of abutment screw loosening or crown cement dissolution.

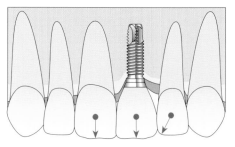

Fig 13-1

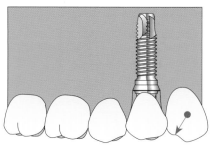

Fig 13-2

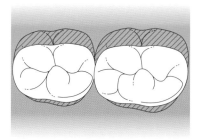

Fig 13-3

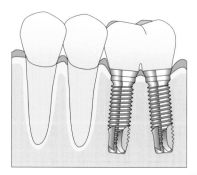

Fig 13-4

Partially Edentulous—
Multiple Units

▼ Posterior Partial Denture

1. Centric contacts should be placed on the posterior fixed partial denture lighter than the natural teeth in casual intercuspation but equal to the natural teeth in maximum intercuspation. Some clinicians will reduce the size of contact on the implant restoration in an attempt to compensate for the lack of periodontal ligament. This can be accomplished at the delivery appointment by adjusting the occlusion, with the patient gently tapping the teeth together. This is followed after the occlusion is adjusted, by having the patient close into the articulating material with maximum occlusal force. Then the clinician reduces the size of the occlusal contacts.[1] The restoration should not be adjusted totally out of occlusion or control of the occlusion will be lost. The potential result (when the implant restoration is taken out of occlusion) is migration of the opposing occlusion and loss of occlusal stability. Interferences in excursive movements may also result.

2. In laterotrusion and protrusion, the ideal is to have no contact on the implant-supported fixed partial denture. (Fig 13–5) This is possible when there is immediate disclusion with a natural canine (mutually protected or cuspid guidance occlusion).

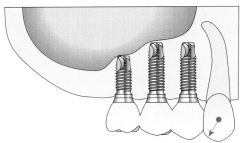

Fig 13-5

13

▼ Anterior Fixed Partial Denture

1. Centric contact should be simultaneous with natural teeth in maximum intercuspation and slightly lighter than the contact of neighboring teeth in casual contact.

2. Often the clinician is forced to place some contact on the prosthetic tooth over the implant on excursive movements. This occurs often when replacing a missing cuspid with an implant-supported fixed partial denture.

3. Some clinicians suggest the goal should be anterior group function. (Fig 13–6)

   a. Attempt to place contact on multiple teeth and over multiple implants if possible.

   b. If the missing canine is replaced by an implant restoration, avoid immediate canine disclusion with all the force on one implant at one time.

   c. Avoid placing all the load on a single implant in excursive movements or in centric contact.

4. Other clinicians would argue that the restoration is a single entity. Force on one portion of the partial denture is distributed to the rest of the partial denture. These clinicians claim that immediate disclusion on one portion of the partial denture is inevitable and of no clinical importance.

5. Still others suggest creating contacts simultaneously on the implant fixed partial denture and natural anterior teeth, in laterotrusive and protrusive movements.

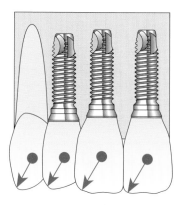

Fig 13-6

Completely Edentulous

▼ Situation (Fig 13–7)

Maxilla: complete denture, no implants

Mandible: complete denture, no implants

1. Nonbalanced occlusion
2. Balanced occlusion
   a. Bilateral balanced-anatomic tooth
   b. Lingualized occlusion
   c. Monoplane-balanced

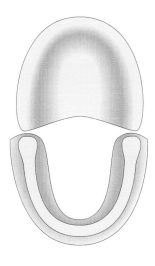

Fig 13-7

▼ Situation (Fig 13–8)

Maxilla: complete denture, no implants

Mandible: overdenture, implants

1. Nonbalanced occlusion
   a. Potential problem with unstable maxillary complete denture
2. Balanced occlusion
   a. Bilateral balanced
   b. Lingualized occlusion
   c. Monoplane-balanced

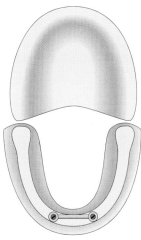

Fig 13-8

▼ Situation (Fig 13–9)

Maxilla: Overdenture, implants

Mandible: Overdenture, implants

1. Nonbalanced occlusion
2. Balanced occlusion
   a. Bilateral balanced
   b. Lingualized occlusion
   c. Monoplane-balanced

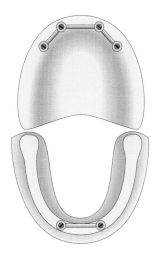

Fig 13-9

13

▼ Situation (Fig 13–10)

Maxilla: complete denture, no implants

Mandible: fixed detachable prosthesis, 4 to 6 implants

1. Nonbalanced occlusion
   a. Potential problem with unstable maxillary complete denture
   b. Potential painful tissue under maxillary complete denture
2. Balanced occlusion
   a. Bilateral balanced
   b. Lingualized

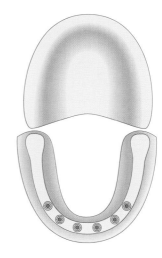

Fig 13-10

▼ Situation (Fig 13–11)

Maxilla: fixed detachable prosthesis, 4 to 6 implants

Mandible: fixed detachable prosthesis, 4 to 6 implants

1. Anterior group function (Fig 13–12)
   a. Simultaneous contact on anterior and posterior teeth in centric—goal is force over the implants. This is often difficult to achieve with a class II malocclusion patient due to lack of anterior occlusal contact.
   b. Contact on multiple teeth and over multiple implants in laterotrusion and protrusion.
   c. No force or contact on cantilever—laterotrusion and protrusion.
   d. Avoid all contact on one tooth or one implant.

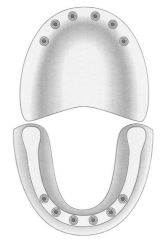

Fig 13-11

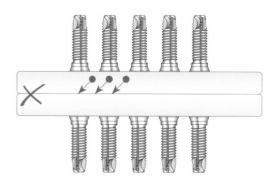

Fig 13-12

Completely and Partially Edentulous

▼ **Situation** (Fig 13–13)

Maxilla: complete denture, no implants

Mandible: dentulous with implant-supported partial denture (teeth + implants)

1. The goal is balanced occlusion (in order to stabilize the maxillary complete denture).
   a. Bilateral balanced
   b. Lingualized occlusion
2. This is difficult to accomplish with natural teeth.

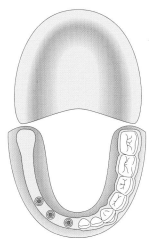

Fig 13-13

▼ **Situation** (Fig 13–14)

Maxilla: overdenture, implants

Mandible: dentulous with implant-supported fixed partial denture (teeth + implants)

1. If the overdenture is totally implant supported, avoid contact in laterotrusion on teeth distal to last implant. It is a cantilever and may place excessive load on the implants.
2. If the overdenture is joint implant and mucosal supported, the goal is bilateral balanced or lingualized occlusion. This is difficult with natural teeth.

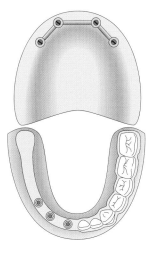

Fig 13-14

13

▼ Situation (Fig 13–15)

Maxilla: fixed detachable prosthesis, implants

Mandible: dentulous with implant-supported fixed partial denture (teeth + implants)

1. In laterotrusion and protrusion, avoid contact on cantilever.
2. In laterotrusion and protrusion, contact is on multiple teeth over multiple implants.
3. Avoid placing all contact on one implant.

Reference

1. Henry P. Osseointegrated implant prosthesis. Presentation to Southern California Dental Association; 1986; Anaheim, CA.

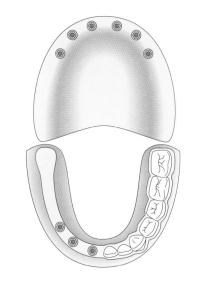

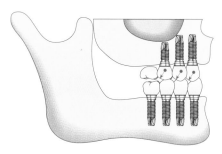

Fig 13-15

Maxillary—Completely Edentulous

Goal

Identify patient's need for a removable or fixed prosthesis. This is critical because a patient's need will dictate the design of the prosthesis and may affect the number of implants placed. For instance if the patient's chief complaint is dislike of the removable aspect of the existing denture, then a fixed prosthesis must be planned. This often includes more implants and careful planning.

Presurgical Needs

1. Mounted diagnostic casts
2. Presurgical wax denture set-up
3. Surgical template
4. Plan for prosthesis type and design, which will determine implant placement
5. Examination of high smile line (which will affect the design and potentially show metal if ignored) without complete denture in
6. Radiographic needs
   a. Panoramic
   b. Lateral cephalometric
   c. Tomogram
   d. Computerized axial tomogram

Considerations

1. The position of the maxillary sinus often prevents posterior implants without additional surgical procedures. (Fig 14–1)

2. Some clinicians consider the edentulous maxilla the most challenging restorative situation for implants.

3. For each patient, the clinician must consider the individual situation, including:

   a. Bone quality

   b. Bone quantity

   c. Maxillo-mandibular relations

   d. Parafunctional habits

   e. Opposing area, occlusion, occlusal material (especially for the edentulous maxilla)

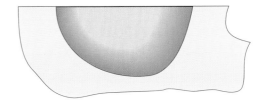

Fig 14-1

Restorative Options[1]

1. Maxillary fixed-detachable prosthesis
(Fig 14–2)

a. **Definition:** An implant-supported prosthesis that is fixed and not removable by the patient. This prosthesis is retrievable by the dentist by unscrewing the retaining screws.

b. **Advantages**
   1. Predictability based on research
   2. Fixedness
   3. Retrievability
   4. No palatal coverage
   5. Usefulness for patients with significant maxillary resorption
   6. The metallic components will not be as likely to show with severe resorption, when combined with a low smile line.

c. **Disadvantages**[1,2]
   1. Maintenance is difficult owing to contours created to hide metal components.
   2. Phonetic problems can result from air escape.
   3. Esthetic problems are possible with short lip or high smile line: the metal components may show.
   4. Limitation on cantilever extension often makes it impossible to match occlusal planes and provide adequate centric contacts with some skeletal relations.
   5. Profile cannot be altered with flange.
   6. The potential site for implants is often only in the anterior maxilla. If the implants end up in a straight line, the cantilever is limited.

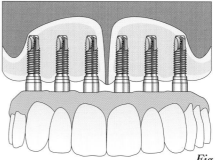

Fig 14-2

14

d. Design considerations

1. Number of implants
   a. At least four
   b. Ideally six or more

2. Design: acrylic-metal restoration (Fig 14–3)

   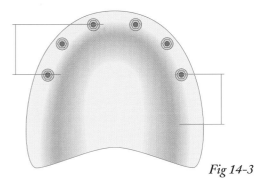

   Fig 14-3

   a. The maximum cantilever length for the acrylic-metal prosthesis is 10 mm. The portion of the partial denture between the most anterior and most distal implants counteracts the lever arm of the cantilever.[3]

   b. If the implants are placed in a straight line, reduce the cantilever. (Fig 14–4)

   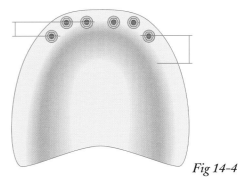

   Fig 14-4

   c. The occlusal gingival height of metal framework should be a minimum of 6 mm to provide rigidity to the prosthesis. (Fig 14–5)

   d. In the maxillary anterior and posterior region, the residual ridge contour results in implants placed with a labial inclination. (Fig 14–6)

   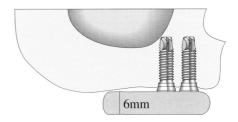

   Fig 14-5

   • The Abutment Selection Kit is helpful for evaluating implant position and angulation. After implant uncovering, an impression can be made to the implant level. A soft-tissue material is used in the region of the implant. Trial abutments are used for diagnostic purposes on the cast.

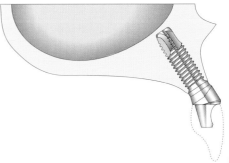

Fig 14-6

- The restorative solution is use of an angulated abutment. The disadvantage is metal show of the angulated abutment or an extension of the prosthesis to cover it. This compromises the patient's ability to practice adequate daily hygiene. A second alternative is a substructure design.

- Because of the difficulty with implant angulation and resulting poor esthetics, some clinicians elect to place the implants in the cuspid and posterior regions. (Fig 14–7)

  The disadvantage is the wide span that results between the cuspids. In some patients, a significant anterior cantilever can result which adds to the force placed on the implants.

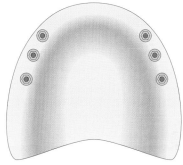

Fig 14-7

e. Prior to the implant placement, special attention should be paid to the maxillo-mandibular relationship.

- Often with the loss of teeth and resorption of the anterior maxilla, the potential implant sites are too far to the palatal of the labial surface of the anterior teeth. The result is a cantilever anterior to the implants and an increased load. (Fig 14–8)

- Some clinicians consider this a reason to consider an implant overdenture as an alternative. Other clinicians may consider surgical options.

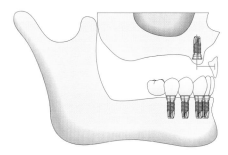

Fig 14-8

14

Design considerations (continued)

3. Design: ceramo-metal restoration (Fig 14–9)

a. Advantages

- Esthetics.

- Opposing a mandibular arch restored with porcelain occlusals results in similar materials contacting.

- In maxillary arch with minimal resorption, a ceramo-metal restoration may be preferred. This option may fit into the limited vertical space and result in better esthetics than other options.

b. Disadvantages

- This technique is technically challenging. It requires a wax try-in of denture teeth with no labial flange and, later, a post-ceramic solder.

- Implant placement is more critical. Implants should be placed in the center of the planned prosthesis to simulate a normal emergence profile.

- With severe vertical resorption, esthetics are compromised due to long prosthetic teeth.

- The resorptive pattern in the maxilla often occurs with the loss of vertical height and loss of labial bone. Fabrication of a ceramo-metal restoration can result in a labial cantilever with severe labial bone loss.

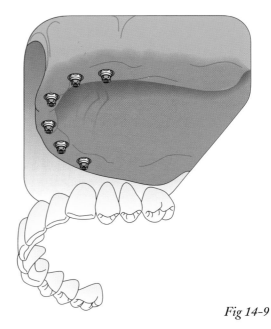

Fig 14-9

- The restoration does not replace missing interdental papilla. This may result in dark triangles between teeth.
- The clinician should remember that as porcelain is baked on the metal framework the shape of the framework changes slightly. This alters the precise fit of the gold cylinder to abutment inter-face. This system works because of a precise fit which is altered by the porcelain application. This error can be reduced by post-ceramic soldering of the restoration, or by making the restoration in several segments.

e. **Maxillo-mandibular relations** (Fig 14–10)

For the completely edentulous maxilla, it is critical to determine the relation of the maxilla to the mandible prior to implant placement. This can be examined with mounted diagnostic casts and a wax try-in denture on a record base. The clinician should note:

- Interarch distance
- Anticipated position of the maxillary anterior teeth in relation to the residual ridge
- How far distal the maxillary occlusal table should extend to provide contacts for the opposing arch

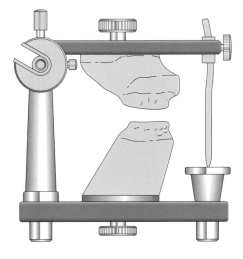

Fig 14-10

14

Maxillo-mandibular relations (continued)

1. Class I Patient: Fixed maxillary prosthesis (Fig 14–11)

   a. Situation: Maxilla completely eden-
      tulous. Class I patient restored with
      a fixed prosthesis on implants in the
      maxilla. Mandible is dentulous.

   b. Goal: Establish simultaneous con-
      tacts with the anterior and poste-
      rior teeth of both arches in maxi-
      mum intercuspal position.

   c. Opposing natural teeth: If the
      mandible is dentulous, the patient
      should have disclusion over the
      implants. Multiple teeth and
      implants should contact on the
      working side. The clinician should
      avoid contact distal to the last
      implant in laterotrusion and protru-
      sion to reduce force on the can-
      tilever. The clinician often has a
      problem extending the cantilever far
      enough distally so that all the nat-
      ural teeth have centric contacts.
      This occurs when mandibular sec-
      ond molars are present.

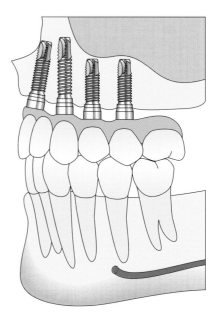

Fig 14-11

2. Class II patient: Fixed maxillary prosthesis (Fig 14–12)

  a. Situation: Class II patients with a completely edentulous maxilla restored with implants and a fixed prosthesis. The mandibular arch is dentulous.

  b. Problem: In a Class II patient with the maxilla anterior to the mandible, there is a problem with matching the occlusal surfaces of the arches and providing adequate occlusal contacts for the mandibular teeth. The implants are often placed in the available bone anterior to the maxillary sinus. The resulting prosthesis cannot be cantilevered more than 10 mm or one tooth distally. The maxilla and the mandible may only contact on one or two teeth per side. If the mandible has natural teeth, centric contacts often cannot be provided for all the natural teeth opposing this prosthesis. Another problem occurs with determining the occlusal scheme. In lateral movements, there will be a significant amount of horizontal force on the cantilevered portion of the maxillary fixed prosthesis. This is because the anterior teeth in some Class II patients do not disclude the posterior teeth immediately.

  c. Solution: The solution is more implants posteriorly and a fixed prosthesis or an overdenture prosthesis that is joint implant/mucosal supported.

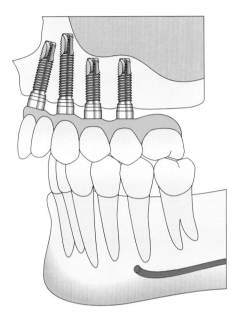

Fig 14-12

14

Maxillo-mandibular relations (continued)

3. Class III patient: Fixed maxillary prosthesis (Fig 14–13)

    a. If implants are vertical, a cantilever forward would result if prosthetic teeth are extended forward to meet the mandibular anteriors.

    b. Implants placed at an angle are desirable for some patients to improve esthetics and allow for centric contacts to occur on the anterior teeth of the prosthesis. (Fig 14–14)

    c. Problem: The result is loading the implants at an angle that is unfavorable with either solution. A lever arm has been created anteriorly and posteriorly, which may potentially overload the implants. (Fig 14–14)

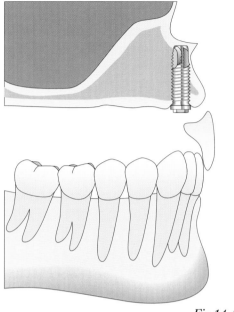

Fig 14-13

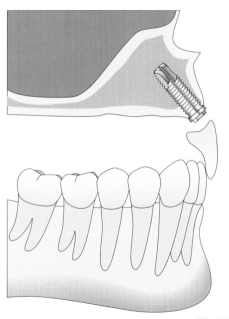

Fig 14-14

2. Maxillary overdenture prosthesis[2,4,5]
(Fig 14–15)

a. Definition: an implant-supported prosthesis that is removable by the patient

b. Advantages
1. Control of profile with a flange
2. Removability
3. East of maintenance
4. Phonetics equivalent to conventional maxillary complete denture
5. Esthetics predictable as metal components covered
6. Useful for severe maxillo-mandibular relations, ie, Class II, Class III
7. Greater technical predictability
8. Greater versatility for more patients

c. Disadvantages
1. Predictability not based on long-term research
2. Removability

d. Considerations
1. Simplify design
   a. Determine if totally implant borne or joint implant/mucosal borne.
   b. Evaluate design as a removable partial denture. The clinician should consider the axis of rotation. When an occlusal load is placed posterior to the axis, the prosthesis rotates. Everything anterior to the axis moves occlusally and everything posterior to the line moves toward the mucosa.

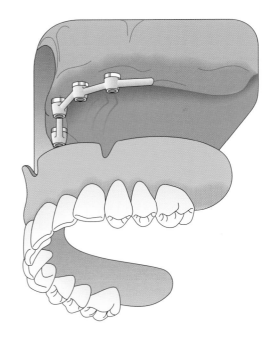

Fig 14-15

14

Maxillary overdenture prosthesis / Considerations (continued)

2. Design: two-implant overdenture

a. Most clinicians will insist on four implants for a maxillary implant-supported overdenture.

b. Improper: two implants (Fig 14–16)

- This design provides no ease of rotation.

- When the occlusal force is on the posterior teeth it causes a bending moment on the bar. The screw joint opens and loosens the screw.

c. Proper: two implants (Fig 14–17)

- This design facilitates rotation of the prosthesis around the bar when loaded.

- The bar should be perpendicular to the midline. Note: many clinicians will insist on four implants for a maxillary implant-supported overdenture.

- Ideally the bar should be a straight line between the implants. Occasionally the bar must be cantilevered anteriorly or posteriorly to stay within the bulkiest part of the prosthesis near the denture teeth. The clinician should keep this cantilever to a minimum.

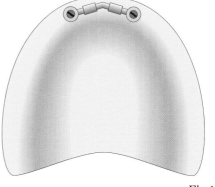

Fig 14-16

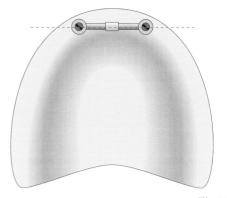

Fig 14-17

3. Design: four-implant overdenture

   a. Joint implant-mucosal–supported prosthesis

      - One clip only in the anterior. (Fig 14–18)

      - Allows ease of rotation. (Fig 14–19)

      - The posterior portion of the denture rotates upward and is supported by the mucosa under the load of mastication.

      - Resilient attachments (ERA, Dalbo) can be added posterior to the most distal gold cylinder. This is still an implant-mucosal–supported prosthesis.

   b. Primarily implant-supported prosthesis (Fig 14–20)

      - No rotation.

      - No fulcrum line.

      - Implant placement: The distance between implants should be wide enough for a clip and two wax or gold connections. Measure the mesiodistal width of the intended clip and add at least 2 to 3 mm for each connector.

      - Need:
        At least 2 mm acrylic over clips;
        Adequate occlusal gingival height of bar or it will flex.

      - The bar should have 6 mm of occlusal gingival height or the cantilever portion of the bar will flex, if the prosthesis is going to be entirely implant supported. (Fig 14–21)

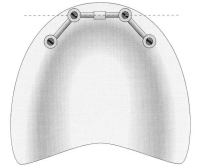

Fig 14-18

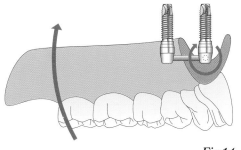

Fig 14-19

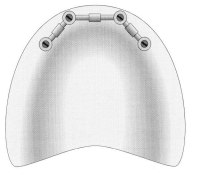

Fig 14-20

14

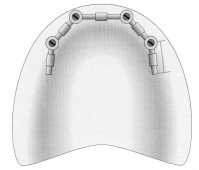

Fig 14-21

Primarily implant-supported prosthesis (continued)

- The length of the cantilever (Fig 14–22) is not the bar length but the length of the occlusal surfaces. Thus, the clinician should measure from the most distal abutment to the distalmost contact to determine the cantilever length.
- Palatal coverage is the first choice. If necessary, the palate can be opened but place the finish line or reinforce inside with metal framework. Usually the palate is opened only if the patient has 6 or more implants. (Fig 14–23)

4. Design: precision-fit overdenture (Fig 14–24)

   a. Overdenture design with an overdenture bar retained by screws can be made by:
   - Wax-up that is surveyed;
   - Framework made via spark-erosion process;
   - Framework made by precision milling.

   b. The overdenture has a metal framework incorporated into it that fits precisely over the bar. The removable overdenture is retained by clips, attachments, or fasteners.

   c. This type of prosthesis has no axis of rotation and is totally implant supported.

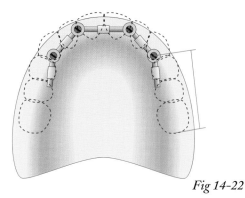

Fig 14-22

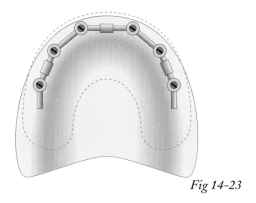

Fig 14-23

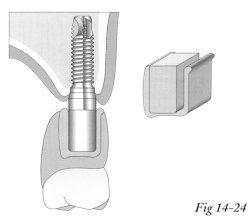

Fig 14-24

5. Design: overdenture with severe maxillary bone loss (Fig 14–25)

a. Situation: Implant placement is only possible in the premolar region due to significant vertical bone loss. This is caused by a lack of adequate vertical height of bone. Many clinicians will not connect the implants of both sides due to the excessive distance anteriorly and across the arch.

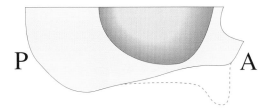

Fig 14-25

- Surgical solution: bone graft
- Restorative options for severe maxillary anterior bone loss (Fig 14–26)

i. Ball attachments. However, avoid this attachment in the maxilla. The ideal solution is more implants and/or grafting.

ii. If four implants are splinted with a bar and clip, the result is a see-saw or first class lever. If the bar is cantilevered far forward, it may exceed the limits of the components. If two implants per side are available, then the implants of each side can be splinted. (Fig 14–27)

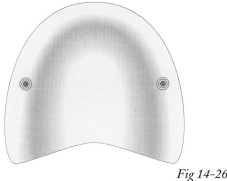

Fig 14-26

The problem is that implants are still only in the molar region and a see-saw or first class lever is the result.

iii. Restorative options include:

- Processed soft liner in the denture area surrounding the bar;
- Attachments with a more universal joint action.

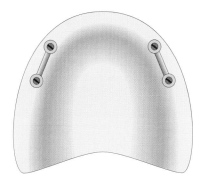

Fig 14-27

14

Design: overdenture with severe maxillary bone loss (continued)

(b) Palatal coverage (Fig 14–28): Many clinicians prefer palatal coverage for a joint implant-mucosal–supported prosthesis. Under the force of mastication, the restoration rotates around the retentive component and loads the mucosa. If the patient requires no palatal coverage, an implant-supported prosthesis should be planned. More implants should also be planned. The definitive implant overdenture should have a palatal finish line or be reinforced with a metal framework.

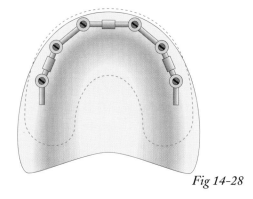

Fig 14-28

Patient Presentations

1. Patient 1

   a. Five osseointegrated implants have been placed in the maxillary completely edentulous arch and a cast gold bar connects all the implants. (Fig 14–29)

   b. A maxillary overdenture has been fabricated over with three retentive clips and an open palate. This prosthesis is totally implant supported. (Fig 14–30)

   c. The patient with maxillary overdenture in place shows the flange, which is useful for altering profile. This flange also stops any air escape that may adversely affect phonetics. The removable aspect of this prosthesis makes it easier for the patient to practice daily oral hygiene. (Fig 14–31)

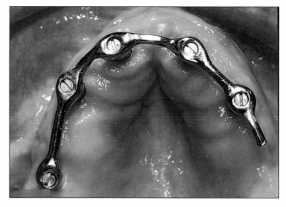

Fig 14-29

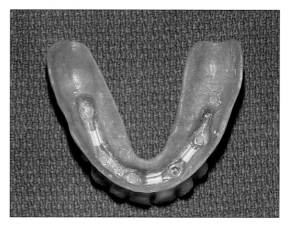

Fig 14-30

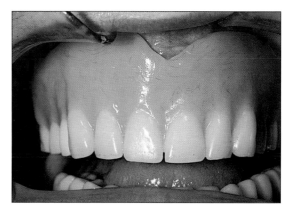

Fig 14-31

Surgery by Dr Peter Moy
Laboratory procedures by Kurt Tennyson

14

2. Patient 2

   a. A completely edentulous maxilla with five osseointegrated implants. A cast gold bar connects the implants with a Hader bar at the midline, and with two ERA attachments cantilevered distally. (Fig 14–32)

   b. The maxillary overdenture with an anterior retentive clip and two ERA attachments. This prosthesis is joint implant and mucosal supported. (Fig 14–33)

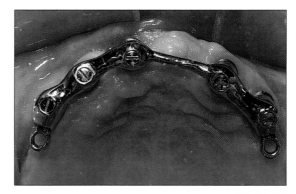

Fig 14-32

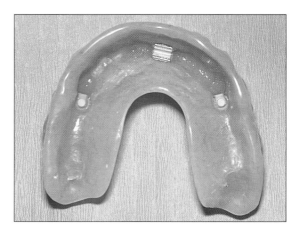

Fig 14-33

Surgery by Dr Richard Martino
Laboratory procedures by Steve Stevens

3. Patient 3

a. A maxillary fixed prosthesis supported by six osseointegrated implants. This is a cast metal framework with denture acrylic and denture teeth. (Fig 14–34)

b. The maxillary fixed detachable prosthesis is supported by six implants. All implants had angulated abutments in place. Note that the width of the maxillary ridge is narrower than where the prosthetic teeth needed to be placed for esthetics and occlusion. This is a result of the resorption of the buccal of the maxillary ridge. (Fig 14–35)

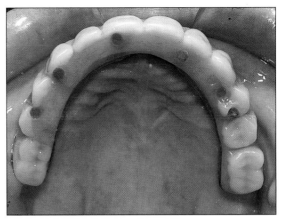

Fig 14-34

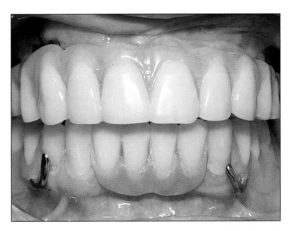

Fig 14-35

14

Surgery by Dr Michael Stohle
Laboratory procedures by Steve Stevens

4. Patient 4

   a. Seven implants were placed in the edentulous maxilla. All the implants had angulated abutments placed but, with the square impression copings and the guide pins in position, an angulation discrepancy can be noted. This is due to the shape of the residual ridge that often occurs in the maxilla. The bone is at an angle in relation to the plane of the occlusion. (Fig 14–36)

   b. Note that implants were placed primarily in the cuspid position and posteriorly. The surgeon elected to do this in order to avoid angulation problems in the anterior region, which can lead to esthetic difficulties. (Fig 14–37)

   c. An anterior view of the restoration shows that the arch size of the prosthetic teeth is significantly larger than the arch size of the edentulous maxilla. This resulted in the entire restoration being cantilevered slightly, buccally and labially to the ridge. Note the ridge lap covering metal components of the restoration. (Fig 14–38)

   d. The anterior smile view shows that the acrylic margin and the metal components are not visible in the high smile of the patient. (Fig 14–39)

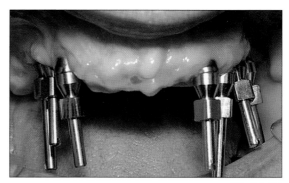

Fig 14-36

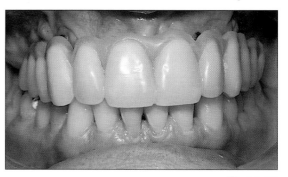

Fig 14-37

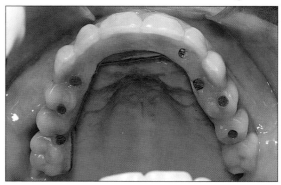

Fig 14-38

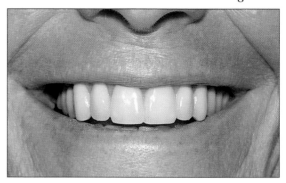

Fig 14-39

Surgery by Dr Burton Becker

Laboratory procedures by Steve Stevens

References

1. Lewis S, Sharma A, Nishimura R. Treatment of edentulous maxilla with osseointegrated implants. J Prosthet Dent 1992;68:503–508.

2. Jemt T, Linden B, Urde G. Failures and complications in 92 consecutively inserted overdentures supported by Brånemark System® implants in severely resorbed edentulous maxillae: A study from prosthetic treatment to first annual check-up. Int J Oral Maxillofac Implants 1992;7:162–167.

3. Rangert B, Jemt T, Jörneus L. Forces and moments on Brånemark implants. Int J Oral Maxillofac Implants 1989;4:241–247.

4. Engquist B, Bergendal T, Kallus T, Linden U. A retrospective multicenter evaluation of osseointegrated implants supporting overdentures. Int J Oral Maxillofac Implants 1988;3:129–134.

5. Engquist B. Overdentures. In: Worthington P, Brånemark PI, eds. Advanced Osseointegration Surgery: Applications in the Maxillofacial Region. Chicago: Quintessence; 1992:233–247.

14

Mandibular—Completely Edentulous

Goal

Determine whether the patient requires fixed or removable prosthesis.

Presurgical Needs

1. Mounted diagnostic casts
2. Wax trial denture set-up
3. Surgical guide
4. Plan for prosthesis type and design, which will determine implant placement
5. Examination of smile line

   If teeth are removed and implants placed soon, there is little resorption of the vertical height of the mandible. There is a potential for metal to show due to this lack of resorption because the restoration and its components will be more superior.

6. Radiographic needs
   a. Panoramic radiograph: essential

   All other radiographic aids utilized if additional information necessary:
   b. Occlusal
   c. Periapicals
   d. Tomograms
   e. Lateral cephalometric
   f. Computerized axial tomograms

Considerations[1]

The mandibular anterior is the most predictable region for implant success.[2]

Restorative Options

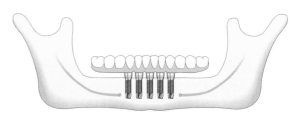

Fig 15-1

1. Fixed partial denture prosthesis: fixed bone-
   anchored partial denture, fixed-detachable
   prosthesis (Fig 15–1)
   a. **Advantages**
      1. Fixedness
      2. Retrievability
      3. Predictability based on research
   b. **Disadvantages**
      1. Limitation on cantilever length
      2. No labial flange, so less profile control
   c. **Number of implants**
      1. Four to six implants, placed between
         mental foramen (Fig 15–2)
      2. For most clinicians, five implants evenly
         spaced in the region

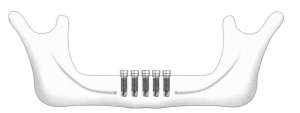

Fig 15-2

   d. **Implant placement—occlusal view**
      1. Implants in a straight line (Fig 15–3)
         The clinician should limit the cantilever
         when all implants are in a straight line.
         There is a significant load on the
         implant components. A bending
         moment on the components may
         result in fracture of the gold screws if
         a fixed prosthesis is made and a can-
         tilever extended. Clinicians will con-
         sider an overdenture for this clinical
         example instead of a fixed detachable
         prosthesis.

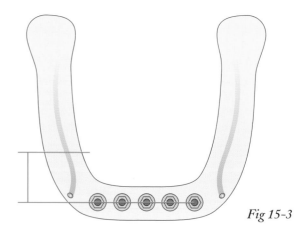

Fig 15-3

2. Implants around a curvature

   With implants around the curvature of the arch (Fig 15–4), the prosthesis can be cantilevered more predictably. The surgeon should attempt to distribute the implants around the curvature of the arch as much as possible. The surgeon should maximize the distance from the anterior to the posterior most implants on each side of the arch.

e. **Implant placement—surgical view** (Fig 15–5)

   Implants are placed by identifying the mental foramen bilaterally and the anterior loop of the nerve which is often 3 mm anterior to the foramen. The surgeon moves anterior to the loop and then places the fixture. The midline follows and then the middle fixture on each side is positioned. Implants (4 mm) are positioned no closer than 7 mm center to center.

f. Cantilever length

   When determining cantilever length the clinician should consider:

   1. Number of fixtures
   2. Placement of fixtures (occlusally)

      When viewed from the occlusal they should not be in a straight line. They should maximize the anterior posterior interfixture distance. Some clinicians use 10 mm as their goal.

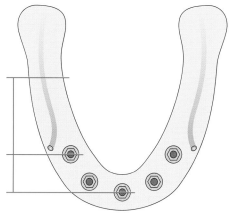

Fig 15-4

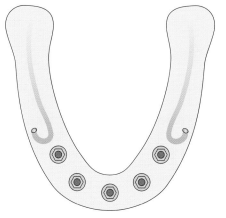

Fig 15-5

15

Cantilever length (continued)

3. Angulation of fixtures

   Fixtures should be placed vertically, or perpendicular to the anticipated occlusal plane. The clinician should be more conservative with the cantilever length when the fixtures are at an angle to the anticipated occlusal plane. The implant components will be loaded at an angle and a greater shear force may result.

4. Length of implants

   Implants of 10 mm or more have been shown to have equivalent success.

5. Bone quality

   Of course, with poor bone quality, the clinician is urged to be more conservative with the restoration.

6. Occlusal force

   The anticipated occlusal force should be considered prior to determining the cantilever length. For patients with a history of parafunctional habits, the clinician should consider shortening the cantilever.

7. Opposing occlusion

   When determining the cantilever length, the clinician should also evaluate the opposing occlusion. A patient with a completely edentulous maxilla may often be cantilevered in the mandible more predictably than a patient with a dentulous maxilla.

8. Cantilever (Figs 15–6a and 15–6b)

There are many methods to determine cantilever length.[3,4] Some clinicians fabricate a maximum cantilever one and a half times the distance from the most anterior to the most posterior abutment. The maximum for the mandible is 20 mm. A 15-year study had patient cantilevers of 16 mm.[2] Another study showed a better survival rate for fixed implant prostheses with cantilevers 15 mm and less.[5]

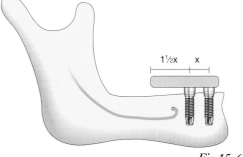

Fig 15-6a

g. Design

Vertical height of metal framework must prevent flexing of metal. (Fig 15–7)

For low-gold, high-palladium alloys, 6 mm of vertical height is necessary.

h. Maxillo-mandibular relations (Fig 15–8)

The relation of the maxilla to the mandible must be evaluated for the potential implant patient with a completely edentulous mandible. This can be done by mounting diagnostic casts and having a wax trial denture fabricated. Prior to surgery, the clinician should evaluate:

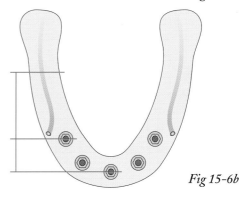

Fig 15-6b

- Interarch distance.
- Relation of the maxillary arch to the mandibular ridge.
- If the maxilla is dentulous, the clinician should determine the proposed cantilever length of the mandibular fixed prosthesis. The clinician should evaluate if an adequate number of maxillary teeth will have centric contacts provided by the mandibular prosthesis.

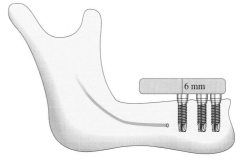

Fig 15-7

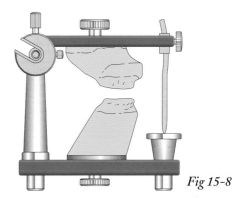

Fig 15-8

15

Maxillo-mandibular relations (continued)

1. Class I patient

   a. For a Class I patient, the maxillo-mandibular relation is ideal. Implants can be placed in a vertical direction and the prosthesis has simultaneous occlusal contacts on all teeth. If the implant prosthesis opposes a maxillary complete denture (Fig 15–9), a bilateral balanced occlusion is often the chosen occlusal scheme. If the implant prosthesis opposes maxillary natural dentition (Fig 15–10), anterior disclusion is the goal. Multiple anterior teeth and multiple implants are in contact in lateral excursions. There is no contact distal to the last implant in lateral movements.

2. Class II patient

   a. If implants are placed in a vertical direction for the Class II patient, centric contacts are often not possible with the anterior prosthetic teeth. If the implant prosthesis opposes natural teeth (Fig 15–11), the clinician should attempt to have laterotrusive contacts only over the implants and no contacts distal to the last implant.

   If the implant prosthesis opposes a maxillary complete denture (Fig 15–12), then a bilateral balanced occlusal scheme should be the goal.

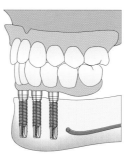

Fig 15-9

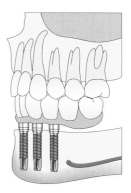

Fig 15-10

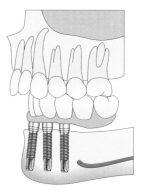

Fig 15-11

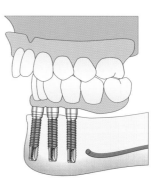

Fig 15-12

b. If the restorative dentist extends the partial denture anteriorly, a lever arm (cantilever) is created and a bending of the prosthesis results. (Fig 15–13) The clinician may also significantly alter the patient's facial profile.

c. Some surgeons attempt to angle the implants anteriorly for a Class II patient. (Fig 15–14) Care should be taken to avoid excessive angulation, which would result in screw access on the facial surface of the prosthetic teeth. The clinician should also remember that an implant placed at an angle is not optimally loaded. Another solution is orthognathic surgery.

3. Class III patient

a. If the surgeon places the implants vertically, then the anterior portion of the prosthesis will either have no centric contacts or will be cantilevered to the lingual. (Fig 15–15)

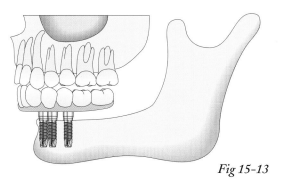

Fig 15-13

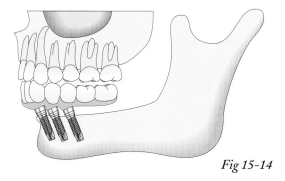

Fig 15-14

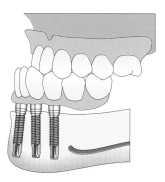

Fig 15-15

15

Maxillo-mandibular relations / Class III patient (continued)

b. For the Class III patient, vertically placed implants are the normal limitation on cantilever length. The restoration may not provide centric contacts for all the maxillary teeth. The result in centric contact is contact primarily in the premolar region with no contact on the maxillary anterior teeth. In lateral excursive movements, forces should be placed over the implants, but this may be difficult because of how the two occlusal planes match up.

c. A second alternative when implants are placed vertically in a Class III patient is to extend the restoration lingually. (Fig 15–16) The restoration becomes a cantilever with an increase in the lever arm, and the screw access holes are often on the facial aspect of the prosthesis. This may interfere with the normal tongue space.

d. A surgical solution for the Class III patient is to angle the implants lingually. (Fig 15–17)

This may sometimes cause abutment emergence close to or in the floor of the mouth, jeopardizing the patient's ability to perform daily oral hygiene.

e. Another solution is orthognathic surgery.

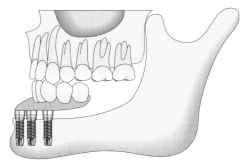

Fig 15-16

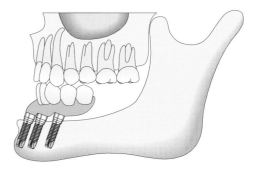

Fig 15-17

2. Overdenture: mandible overdenture[6]

a. Bar shape (cross-section) (Fig 15–18)

1. Circular—allows rotation
2. Circular and extension—allows rotation
3. Ovoid (avoid)

b. Two implants

1. Two implants plus clip—basic design[7]

   a. The bar should be perpendicular to midline. (Fig 15–19)

   The result is a clip that rotates easily around the bar (ease of rotation). (Fig 15–20)

   This prosthesis is joint implant-mucosal supported.

   b. The bar should be parallel to a line drawn through retromolar pad midlines. (Fig 15–21)

   The result is ease of rotation around the bar.

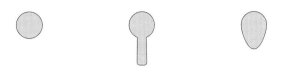

Fig 15-18

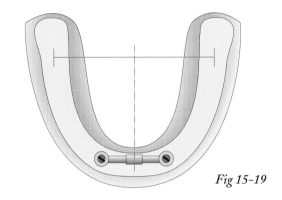

Fig 15-19

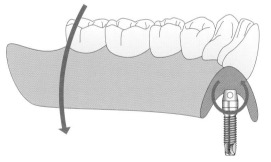

Fig 15-20

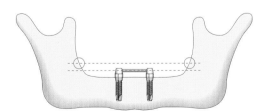

Fig 15-21

15

Two implants plus clip—basic design (continued)

- The bar will be parallel to the retromolar-pad midline at varying heights above the soft tissue, depending on the amount of resorption. (Fig 15–22)

c. If the clinician plans placement of two implants, all potential implant sites should be identified and marked. (Fig 15–23)

The sites are identified as 1 to 5 between the mental foramen. Implants should be placed in positions 2 and 4 if possible. This allows for implant placement in sites 1, 3, and 5 in the future if the patient requires it. Thus, the clinician has assured convertibility from an overdenture to a fixed partial denture.

d. Advantages (Fig 15–24)

- Joint implant-mucosal borne
- Ease of rotation
- Two implants with bar attachments utilized on bar and attachments
- Ideal

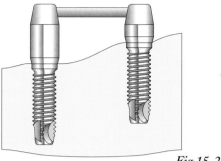
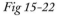

Fig 15-22

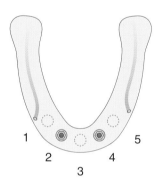

Fig 15-23

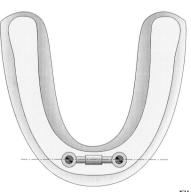

Fig 15-24

2. Two implants with bar and clip plus two attachments (distal) (Fig 15–25)

   a. Disadvantage
      - Axis of rotation moved posterior
      - A cantilever exists distal to gold cylinder
      - Two fulcrum lines or axes of rotation
      - Potential opening of screw joint and loosening of screw because design has prevented ease of rotation and has locked on the bar
      - Possible fracture of the attachment

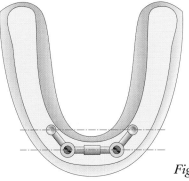

Fig 15-25

3. Two implants and distal attachments only, without clip (Fig 15–26)

   a. Advantage
      - Ease of rotation

   b. Disadvantages
      - Fulcrum line more posterior
      - Possible increase anterior vertical movement of the prosthesis
      - See-saw created
      - Fracture of the attachments off of the bar
      - Loosen screws or fracture

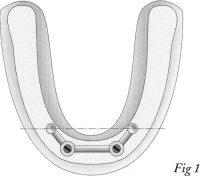

Fig 15-26

c. Three implants (Fig 15–27)

   1. Three implants and ball attachment

      a. Useful if three implants placed, as it is difficult to place bar and clip in anterior region with three implants.

      b. Some clinicians report loosening of the abutment screws with taller abutment heights when the ball attachments are used.

      c. O-ring retainer in the complete denture is wide buccolingually. Some complete dentures will be unable to accommodate it.

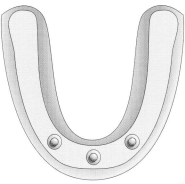

Fig 15-27

15

Three implants and ball-attachment (continued)

2. Three implants and bar (Fig 15–28)

a. Restoring with one clip allows for rotation.

b. Restoring with multiple clips or clips and attachments creates an overdenture that is totally implant supported and not joint implant-mucosal borne. (Fig 15–29)

Avoid this option, which risks loosening of screws or fracture of attachments.

c. If implants are placed in positions 1, 3, and 5, it is often difficult to achieve ease of rotation of the prosthesis with a bar and clip attachment. This option does not allow for rotation of the clip around the bar. The three implants in this situation are primarily supporting the entire prosthesis. (Fig 15–30)

Avoid this design. One alternative is to omit the clips, letting the attachments extended posteriorly retain the denture.

d. Another alternative is to position the bar so that the clips and the bar are perpendicular to the midline of the arch. Clips can then be placed on either side of the middle implant. The problem is that the prosthesis may interfere with tongue space.

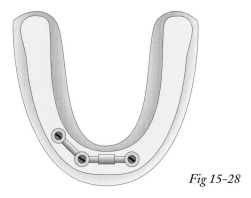

Fig 15-28

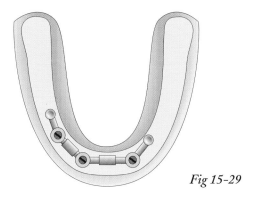

Fig 15-29

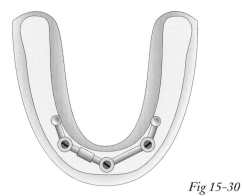

Fig 15-30

d. Four implants (Figs 15–31 and 15–32)

  1. Four implants and bar with one clip

    a. Advantages

      • Ease of rotation

      • Joint implant-mucosal borne

  2. Four implants, bar and multiple clips (Fig 15–33)

    a. Advantages

      • Totally implant-borne prosthesis

      • Increased retention

      • Increased stability

      • Removability by patient

    b. Disadvantages

      • Implants support full occlusal force.

      • Why not fabricate a fixed prosthesis?

  3. Four implants, bar, cantilevers and multiple clips (Fig 15–34)

    a. Advantages

      • Totally implant-supported prosthesis. The clinician must limit the cantilever length to restore. The occlusal gingival height of the bar should be 6 mm for rigidity.

      • This prosthesis is similar in function to the fixed-detachable prosthesis.

    b. Disadvantages

      • Fracture of cantilevered bar distal to the distal-most gold cylinder. This occurs if the bar has inadequate occlusogingival height or the cantilever is too long.

      • Why not fabricate a fixed prosthesis?

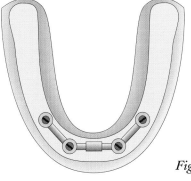

Fig 15-31

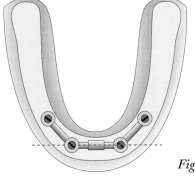

Fig 15-32

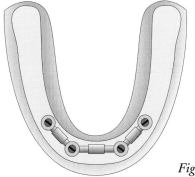

Fig 15-33

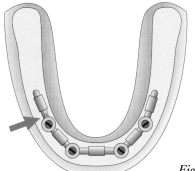

Fig 15-34

15

Four implants, bar, cantilever, and multiple clip (continued)

c. Design considerations (Fig 15–35)

- Occlusal gingival height of the bar should be 6 mm as this functions much like a fixed prosthesis.

- Cantilever length should be measured from the distal edge of the last gold cylinder to the distal edge of the last tooth. The length of the occlusal table determines the actual cantilever length, not the length of the bar. The clinician should measure the anterior-posterior interfixture distance of the implants, multiplying by 1.5 or 2 for the cantilever limitation. The cantilever length is calculated as if it were a fixed prosthesis.

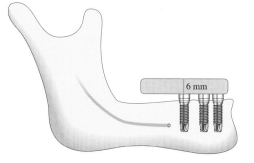

Fig 15-35

Patient Presentations

1. Patient 1
   a. A cast gold Hader bar is used to splint two osseointegrated implants. (Fig 15–36)
   b. The overdenture has a single retentive clip in the anterior portion. This clip is in the midline due to the position of the bar, which allows easy rotation around this bar and the prosthesis. (Fig 15–37)

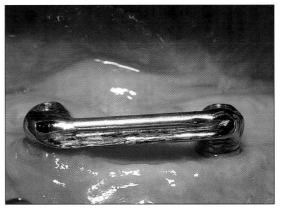

Fig 15-36

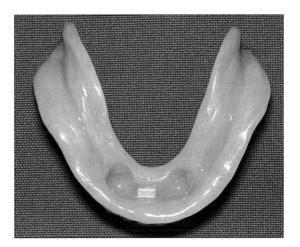

Fig 15-37

Surgery by Dr Peter Moy
Laboratory procedures by Wayne Mito

15

2. Patient 2

   a. Occlusal view of a mandibular fixed-detachable prosthesis shows an optimal anterior posterior spread of the osseointegrated implants. The placement of the five implants enables this patient to be restored with a cantilever that is predictable. (Fig 15–38)

   b. Fixed prosthesis of the same patient opposing a maxillary complete denture. Notice that the metal framework is kept several millimeters above the soft tissue to allow ease of cleaning. (Fig 15–39)

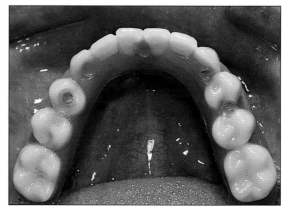

Fig 15-38

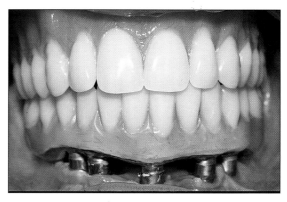

Fig 15-39

Surgery by Dr Todd Jensen
Laboratory procedures by Steve Stevens

References

1. Rangert B, Jemt T, Jörneus L. Forces and moments in Brånemark implants. Int J Oral Maxillofac Implants 1989;4:241–247.

2. Adell R, Lekholm B, Rockler, Brånemark PI. A 15-year study of osseointegrated implants in the treatment of the edentulous jaw. Int J Oral Surg 1981;10:387–416.

3. Rodriguez A, Aquilino S, Lund P. Cantilever length and implant biomechanics: A review of the literature, Part 1. J Prosthod 1994;3:41–46

4. Rodriguez A, Aquilino S, Lund P. Cantilever length and implant biomechanics: A review of the literature, Part 2. J Prosthod 1994;3:114–118

5. Shackleton J, Carr L, Slabbert J, Becker P. Survival length of fixed implant-supported prostheses related to cantilever lengths. J Prosthet Dent 1994;71:23–26.

6. Engquist B. Overdentures. In: Worthington P, Brånemark PI, eds. Advanced Osseointegration Surgery: Applications in the Maxillofacial Region. Chicago: Quintessence; 1992;233–247.

7. Beumer J, Lewis S. The Brånemark Implant System: Clinical and Laboratory Procedures. St. Louis: Ishyaku Euroamerica, 1989.

Prosthodontic Procedure Flowsheets

The restoration of each patient is unique. However, there are many similarities in treatment of patients. The following outlines are included to assist the restorative dentist in planning the actual treatment. Clinical appointments and laboratory procedures are shown in outline form so that the restorative dentist can easily refer to these and follow along with the patient's treatment. There will be many alterations to the suggested flow of treatment due to the unique protocol followed by each dentist, laboratory technician, or surgeon. These outlines are included and are to assist the treatment of the partially edentulous and completely edentulous patients.

Fixed Partial Denture Supported by Osseointegrated Implants

Those procedures in parentheses are optional or not necessary with every patient example.

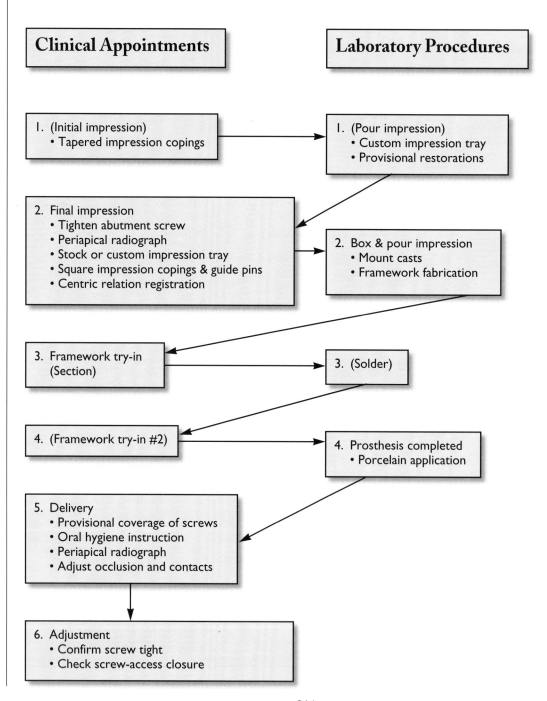

Clinical Appointments

1. (Initial impression)
   • Tapered impression copings

2. Final impression
   • Tighten abutment screw
   • Periapical radiograph
   • Stock or custom impression tray
   • Square impression copings & guide pins
   • Centric relation registration

3. Framework try-in
   (Section)

4. (Framework try-in #2)

5. Delivery
   • Provisional coverage of screws
   • Oral hygiene instruction
   • Periapical radiograph
   • Adjust occlusion and contacts

6. Adjustment
   • Confirm screw tight
   • Check screw-access closure

Laboratory Procedures

1. (Pour impression)
   • Custom impression tray
   • Provisional restorations

2. Box & pour impression
   • Mount casts
   • Framework fabrication

3. (Solder)

4. Prosthesis completed
   • Porcelain application

Overdenture Supported by Osseointegrated Implants— for Two Implants

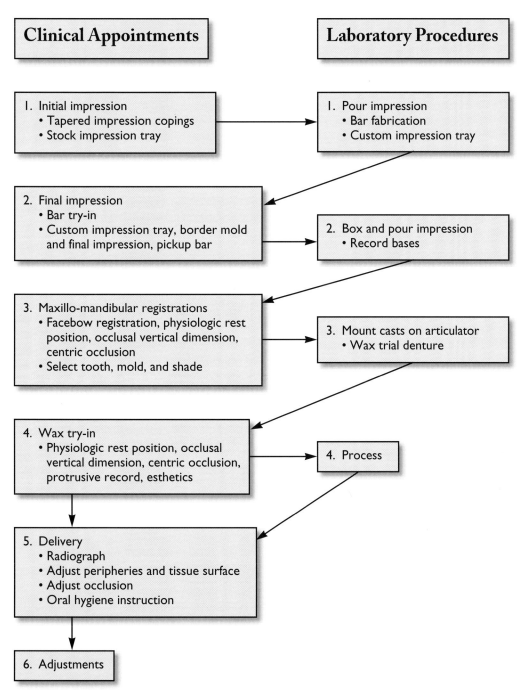

Clinical Appointments

1. Initial impression
   • Tapered impression copings
   • Stock impression tray

2. Final impression
   • Bar try-in
   • Custom impression tray, border mold and final impression, pickup bar

3. Maxillo-mandibular registrations
   • Facebow registration, physiologic rest position, occlusal vertical dimension, centric occlusion
   • Select tooth, mold, and shade

4. Wax try-in
   • Physiologic rest position, occlusal vertical dimension, centric occlusion, protrusive record, esthetics

5. Delivery
   • Radiograph
   • Adjust peripheries and tissue surface
   • Adjust occlusion
   • Oral hygiene instruction

6. Adjustments

Laboratory Procedures

1. Pour impression
   • Bar fabrication
   • Custom impression tray

2. Box and pour impression
   • Record bases

3. Mount casts on articulator
   • Wax trial denture

4. Process

16

Overdenture Supported by Osseointegrated Implants— for Two or More Implants

Those procedures in parentheses are optional or not necessary with every patient example.

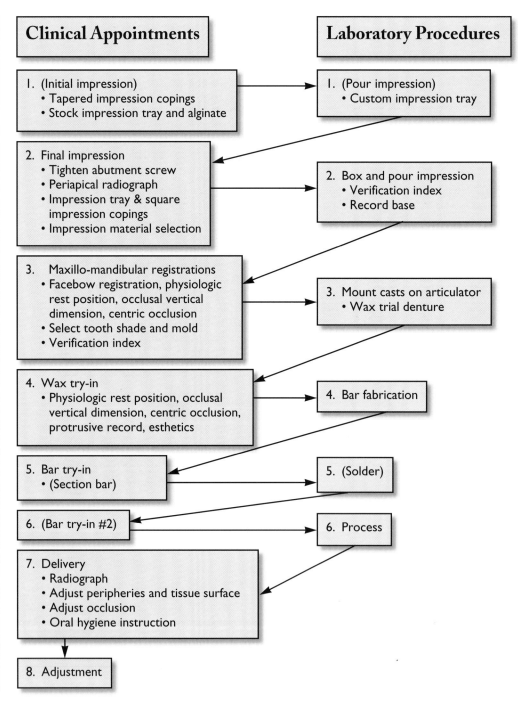

Clinical Appointments

1. (Initial impression)
   - Tapered impression copings
   - Stock impression tray and alginate

2. Final impression
   - Tighten abutment screw
   - Periapical radiograph
   - Impression tray & square impression copings
   - Impression material selection

3. Maxillo-mandibular registrations
   - Facebow registration, physiologic rest position, occlusal vertical dimension, centric occlusion
   - Select tooth shade and mold
   - Verification index

4. Wax try-in
   - Physiologic rest position, occlusal vertical dimension, centric occlusion, protrusive record, esthetics

5. Bar try-in
   - (Section bar)

6. (Bar try-in #2)

7. Delivery
   - Radiograph
   - Adjust peripheries and tissue surface
   - Adjust occlusion
   - Oral hygiene instruction

8. Adjustment

Laboratory Procedures

1. (Pour impression)
   - Custom impression tray

2. Box and pour impression
   - Verification index
   - Record base

3. Mount casts on articulator
   - Wax trial denture

4. Bar fabrication

5. (Solder)

6. Process

218
▼

Fixed Detachable Prosthesis for Completely Edentulous Patient

Those procedures in parentheses are optional or not necessary with every patient example.

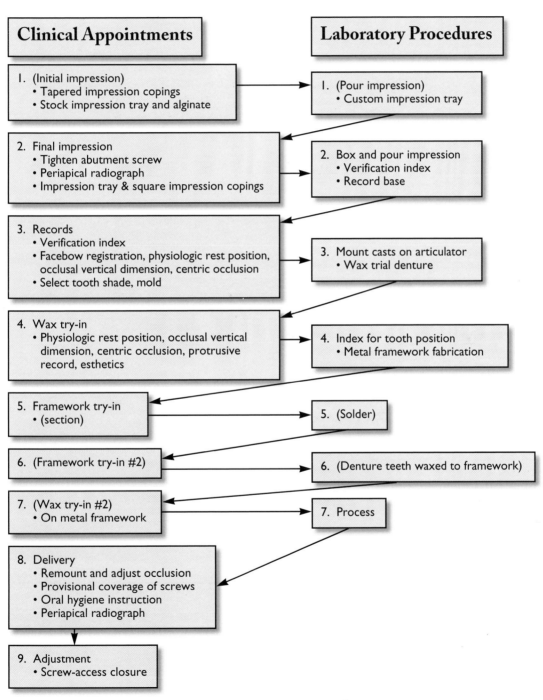

Clinical Appointments

1. (Initial impression)
   - Tapered impression copings
   - Stock impression tray and alginate

2. Final impression
   - Tighten abutment screw
   - Periapical radiograph
   - Impression tray & square impression copings

3. Records
   - Verification index
   - Facebow registration, physiologic rest position, occlusal vertical dimension, centric occlusion
   - Select tooth shade, mold

4. Wax try-in
   - Physiologic rest position, occlusal vertical dimension, centric occlusion, protrusive record, esthetics

5. Framework try-in
   - (section)

6. (Framework try-in #2)

7. (Wax try-in #2)
   - On metal framework

8. Delivery
   - Remount and adjust occlusion
   - Provisional coverage of screws
   - Oral hygiene instruction
   - Periapical radiograph

9. Adjustment
   - Screw-access closure

Laboratory Procedures

1. (Pour impression)
   - Custom impression tray

2. Box and pour impression
   - Verification index
   - Record base

3. Mount casts on articulator
   - Wax trial denture

4. Index for tooth position
   - Metal framework fabrication

5. (Solder)

6. (Denture teeth waxed to framework)

7. Process

16